MW00711087

# Psychosocial Crises

Springhouse Corporation
Springhouse, Pennsylvania

# STAFF

**Executive Director, Editorial**
Stanley Loeb

**Editorial Director**
Matthew Cahill

**Clinical Director**
Barbara F. McVan, RN

**Art Director**
John Hubbard

**Senior Editor**
William J. Kelly

**Clinical Project Editor**
Joanne Patzek DaCunha, RN, BS

**Editors**
Marylou Ambrose, Stephen Daly, Margaret Eckman, Kevin Law, Elizabeth Mauro

**Clinical Editors**
Mary C. Gyetvan, RN, BSEd; Joan E. Mason, RN, EdM; Judith A. Schilling McCann, RN, BSN; Susan Gatzert-Snyder, RN, MS, CS; Beverly Ann Tscheschlog, RN; Steven J. Schweon. RN, BSN

**Copy Editors**
Jane V. Cray (supervisor), Nancy Papsin, Doris Weinstock

**Designers**
Stephanie Peters (associate art director), Matie Patterson (senior designer), Linda Franklin

**Illustrators**
Dimitrios Bastas, Robert Jackson, Robert Neumann, Judy Newhouse, Robert Phillips, Dennis Schofield

**Art Production**
Robert Perry (manager), Donald Knauss, Thomas Robbins, Robert Wieder

**Typography**
David Kosten (director), Diane Paluba (manager), Elizabeth Bergman, Joyce Rossi Biletz, Phyllis Marron, Robin Rantz, Valerie Rosenberger

**Manufacturing**
Deborah Meiris (manager), T.A. Landis, Jennifer Suter

**Production Coordination**
Colleen M. Hayman

**Editorial Assistants**
Maree DeRosa, Beverly Lane, Mary Madden

CS10-020792

Library of Congress Cataloging-in-Publication Data
**Psychosocial crises.**
    p. cm. – (Clinical Skillbuilders™)
    Includes bibliographical references and index.
    1. Psychiatric nursing.    2. Crisis intervention (Psychiatry)
I. Springhouse Corporation.    II. Series.
    [DNLM:   1. Adaptation, Psychological – nurses' instruction.   2. Crisis Intervention – nurses' instruction.   3. Social Alienation – psychology – nurses' instruction.   4. Stress, Psychological – nurses' instruction.   WM 401 P9743]
RC440.P775      1992
610.73 – dc20
DNLM/DLC                                              91-5159
ISBN 0-87434-482-4                                       CIP

# CONTENTS

Advisory board    **iv**

Contributors    **v**

Foreword    **vii**

CHAPTER 1
**Fundamental concepts**    **1**

CHAPTER 2
**Assessment**    **18**

CHAPTER 3
**Behavioral problems**    **32**

CHAPTER 4
**Anxiety**    **60**

CHAPTER 5
**Confusion**    **78**

CHAPTER 6
**Depression**    **90**

CHAPTER 7
**Grief**    **110**

CHAPTER 8
**Schizophrenia and other psychotic disorders**    **122**

CHAPTER 9
**Eating disorders and obesity**    **140**

CHAPTER 10
**Child, spouse, and elder abuse**    **162**

CHAPTER 11
**Substance abuse**    **185**

**Self-test**    **208**

**Index**    **212**

## ADVISORY BOARD

# CONTRIBUTORS

At the time of publication, the contributors held the following positions.

**Joan M. Baker, RN, MS, CS**
Clinical Nurse Specialist, Adult Psychiatry and Mental Health
University of Washington Medical Center
Seattle

**Mary Ann Barbee, RN, MS**
Assistant Executive Director, Clinical Services
Cedar Springs Psychiatric Hospital
Colorado Springs, Colo.

**Jocelyn M. Barr, RN,C, BS**
Nurse Manager, Mental Health Unit
Montgomery Hospital
Norristown, Pa.

**Cornelia M. Beck, RN, PhD**
Associate Dean for Research and Evaluation
University of Arkansas for Medical Sciences
College of Nursing
Little Rock, Ark.

**Elissa Brown, RN, MSN, CS**
Clinical Nurse Specialist, Psychiatry and Mental Health
Veterans Administration Medical Center
Sepulveda, Calif.

**Robert E. Cosgray, RN,C, MA**
Director of Nursing
Logansport (Ind.) State Hospital

**Mary Helen Davis, MD**
Associate Clinical Director
Norton Psychiatric Clinic
Assistant Professor
Department of Psychiatry and Behavioral Sciences
University of Louisville (Ky.) School of Medicine

**Jane Dunn, RN, MSN, CNAA**
Director, Psychiatric Services
Northwest Community Hospital
Arlington Heights, Ill.

**Christine Fitzpatrick, RN, MSN**
Director of Staff Education
Erich Lindemann Mental Health Center
Boston

**Susan Gatzert-Snyder, RN, MS, CS**
Staff Nurse
Northwestern Institute
Fort Washington, Pa.

**Vickie M. Hanna, RN**
Nurse Supervisor, Men's Treatment Unit
Logansport (Ind.) State Hospital

**Alene Harrison, RN, EdD**
Chairperson
Department of Nursing
Idaho State University
Pocatello, Idaho

**Gail Levy, RN, MS, CS**
Psychiatric Clinical Nurse Specialist
Massachusetts General Hospital
Boston

**Teresa A. Palmer, RN,C, MSN, ANP**
Nurse Practitioner
University of Medicine and Dentistry Community Health Center at Piscataway (N.J.)

**Anthony J. Pignone, RN, BSN**
Head Nurse, Manager
Massachusetts General Hospital
Boston

**Ruth P. Rawlins, RN, DSN, CS**
Assistant Professor
University of Arkansas for Medical Sciences
Little Rock, Ark.

**Linda E. Reese, RN, MA**
Deputy Chairperson, Department of Nursing
Assistant Professor
College of Staten Island (N.Y.)

**Frances Schwartz, RN, EdD**
Nurse Educator
Franklin D. Roosevelt Veterans Administration Hospital
Montrose, N.Y.

**Roberta Schweitzer, RN, MSN, CS**
Private Practitioner, Psychodramatics
Nursing Consultant
Phoenix, Ariz.

**Jerilyn Arone Smith, RN,C**
Nurse Educator, Staff Growth and Development
Logansport (Ind.) State Hospital

**Michelle L. Spurlock, RN, BSN**
Nurse Manager, Adult Psychiatry
Norton Psychiatric Clinic
Louisville, Ky.

**Sharon Valente, RN, PhD, CS, FAAN**
Assistant Professor
University of Southern California
Los Angeles

**Karen Goyette Vincent, RN, MS, CS**
Psychiatric Clinical Nurse Specialist
Brockton-West Roxbury Veterans Administration Medical Center
Brockton, Mass.

# FOREWORD

Severe anxiety. Depression. Anorexia nervosa. Substance abuse. You may not immediately associate these problems with medical-surgical or critical care units. But if you work in these areas of the hospital, you undoubtedly see patients with such psychosocial crises everyday.

For some patients, a psychosocial crisis results directly from a physical problem—when a myocardial infarction triggers depression, for instance. For others, the stress of hospitalization may exacerbate a preexisting condition, such as a behavioral problem. For still others, the psychosocial crisis itself leads to hospitalization—for example, when a patient has been physically abused.

But no matter what the cause of the psychosocial crisis, the patient needs your help to deal with it effectively. To help him, you must first know how to recognize the signs of such a crisis. Then you must know how to assess the patient, initiate appropriate interventions, and evaluate the success of those interventions. You also need to know when to request a psychiatric consultation.

*Psychosocial Crises,* the latest volume in the Clinical Skillbuilders series, gives you all this information and more. Written for nurses who deal primarily with physical problems, this compact volume is filled with valuable information on helping patients cope with a variety of psychosocial crises.

The book begins with a chapter on fundamental concepts, including how stress triggers psychosocial crises. The second chapter guides you through the assessment process, explaining everything from using the best communication techniques to evaluating a patient's mental status.

Chapters 3 through 11 focus on the specific types of psychosocial crises you're likely to face. To make your job easier, each chapter follows the same format—first giving you an overview of each problem, then explaining how to assess, intervene, and evaluate.

In Chapter 3, you'll read about behavioral problems, including manipulation, noncompliance, aggression, inappropriate sexual behavior, malingering, obsessive-compulsive behavior, and dependency. Chapter 4 covers anxiety, pointing out ways to help a patient whose problem is so severe that it interferes with your care—and his recovery. Chapter 5 distinguishes between the two major causes of confusion—delirium and dementia—then tells you how to care for confused patients. Chapter 6 covers depressed patients, while Chapter 7 focuses on grieving patients and family members.

In Chapter 8, you'll read about how to help patients with schizophrenia and other psychotic disorders. The next chapter focuses on anorexia, bulimia, and obesity. Chapter 10 helps you recognize the signs of child, spouse, and elder abuse and provides guidelines for giving abused patients the sensitive care they need. You'll also find information on the legal issues that surround abuse. In the final chapter, you'll read about caring for patients who have drug and alcohol problems.

Throughout the book, special graphic devices called logos highlight certain recurring themes. When you see an *Urgent intervention* logo, you'll find a description of actions you should take to quickly help a patient or deal with a potentially dangerous situation—when a violent patient has a weapon, for instance. An *Assessment tip* logo indicates special tips or techniques you can use to evaluate a patient's condition. In Chapter 6, this logo accompanies a sidebar on how to assess your patient's risk of suicide. And a *Checklist* logo signals a list of important points to remember, such as the characteristics of an abusive parent.

Following the last chapter, you'll find a multiple-choice self-test, complete with answers at the end. Taking this test will help you sharpen your skills and assess how much you've learned.

In short, *Psychosocial Crises* is a special book that fills a special need. It provides a world of practical and valuable information to nurses who aren't psychiatric specialists but who must deal with patients in psychosocial crises everyday. And it presents this information clearly and concisely—in plain English. In my opinion, these characteristics make *Psychosocial Crises* an essential resource. I highly recommend it for any nurse who cares for patients.

Grayce M. Sills, RN, PhD, FAAN
Professor Emeritus
Ohio State University
Columbus, Ohio
Chair, Study Committee on Mental Health
Services, State of Ohio

# 1

# FUNDAMENTAL CONCEPTS

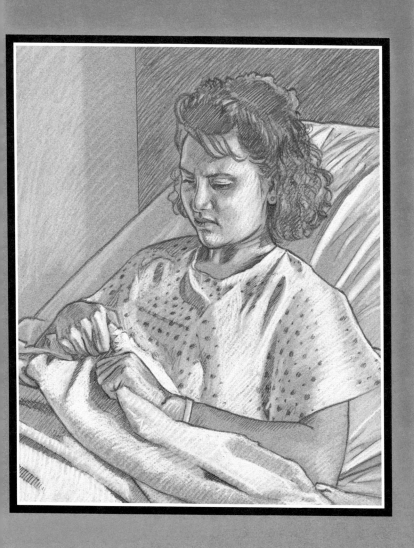

When you enter the room of Mrs. Sanchez, a 55-year-old mastectomy patient, you notice that she's silently staring out the window. She has hardly touched her lunch and doesn't respond when you gently ask if she wants to eat any more. She's clearly troubled — probably by the mastectomy, perhaps by other family problems too.

Every day, you care for patients like Mrs. Sanchez, patients whose psychosocial problems interfere with their recovery. And, as a nurse, you're in the best position to detect such problems early and intervene to alleviate or resolve them — before a psychosocial crisis develops.

Typically, psychosocial problems stem from increased stress produced by a real or perceived threat to a person's physical or psychological well-being. Such stress usually arises from emotional, behavioral, interpersonal, or spiritual conflicts. But hospitalization and illness can also produce stress, either causing or exacerbating psychosocial problems. (See *Stress in the hospitalized patient.*)

When faced with increased stress, a patient will respond by using coping mechanisms that have worked in the past. Mrs. Sanchez, for example, withdraws into silence. But even if such mechanisms help a patient adapt, they may not help him adapt well. And when a patient's behavior is maladaptive, not only will the underlying problem continue, but new problems may develop.

Such a patient needs your help to develop more effective coping skills. By listening carefully to him and assessing his ability to cope, you can help him develop such skills so that he can become as healthy and independent as possible. (See *Psychosocial crises versus mental illness,* page 4.)

This chapter will help you understand the nature of stress, including its physiologic and psychological effects. You'll also review some important theories on the stress response. Next, you'll read about how a patient copes with stress and how a psychosocial crisis can develop when he doesn't cope successfully. After that, you'll find theories explaining the phases of a crisis. Then come guidelines for assessing your patient, setting realistic goals, intervening to help him, and evaluating his progress. Finally, the chapter examines some of the legal issues surrounding the treatment of patients in psychosocial crisis.

# Understanding stress

Stress doesn't automatically lead to psychosocial problems. In fact, a person needs some stress to function normally. But when a person experiences more stress than he can handle, damaging physiologic and psychological changes can result.

## Effects of stress
Physiologic changes brought on by stress may include increased heart rate, headaches, fatigue, stomachaches, sleep disturbances, changes in appetite, and ulcers. Psychological changes include mood swings, irritability, depression, withdrawal, anger, forgetfulness, lack of interest, and an inability to concentrate or to feel pleasure. Stress can also cause a person to question his spiritual beliefs.

Because of the intricate connection between body and mind, psychological stress leads to physiologic stress, and vice versa. Rage, for instance, stimulates the sympathetic

## Stress in the hospitalized patient

The stress caused by a patient's illness and hospitalization, compounded by any underlying stress, can trigger a psychosocial crisis. Below, you'll find a list of stressors that commonly affect hospitalized patients.

☐ *Sense of danger.* Illness and hospitalization can provoke fear, especially fear of the unknown, and threaten the patient's self-image.

☐ *Information overload.* Receiving too much information, particularly when the patient is already feeling anxious, can cause stress.

☐ *Uncertainty and understimulation.* The sensory deprivation or boredom that illness and hospitalization can cause — plus the anxiety of being in a hospital — can trigger stress.

☐ *Ego-control failure.* The patient feels powerless when he's ill. He must depend on others for help.

☐ *Ego-mastery failure.* This occurs when the patient tries to overcome his feelings of powerlessness — perhaps by learning more about his illness and treatment — and his efforts meet with little or no success. He feels stress even more intensely after this failure.

☐ *Threat to self-esteem.* The more threatening the illness, the more a patient's self-esteem is affected — and the more stress he feels.

☐ *Fear of losing respect.* Stress may result from the patient's sense that he's a burden to others and that he'll eventually lose their respect and be abandoned.

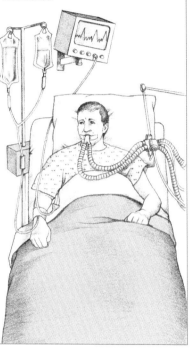

branch of the autonomic nervous system, triggering the fight-or-flight response. A soothing emotion affects the parasympathetic branch, resulting in relaxation. Psychological stimuli may also suppress or stimulate the immune system by affecting neurotransmitter levels.

### Explaining the stress response

Several theories attempt to explain the stress response. They include the general adaptation syndrome theory, Lazarus's theory, Holmes and Rahe's theory, the general systems theory, Freud's intrapsychic theory, the cognitive theory, and the interpersonal theory.

***General adaptation syndrome theory.*** Hans Selye's general adaptation syndrome theory explains a person's organized response to stress. According to the theory, three stress-response stages occur.

In the *alarm stage,* the person

## Psychosocial crises versus mental illness

A mentally healthy person is someone who typically maintains a state of emotional equilibrium—someone who's comfortable with himself and who can use resources constructively and function well within a defined society.

This describes most people who experience psychosocial crises. They are *not* mentally ill. They're mentally healthy people who are temporarily experiencing extreme stress. Remember, only about 10% to 15% of the population have some type of mental illness, but nearly everyone will experience a psychosocial problem at some time.

tries to adjust to a stressor he consciously or unconsciously perceives as threatening. His autonomic nervous system initiates the lifesaving fight-or-flight response. In the *resistance stage*, the person maintains a greater-than-normal resistance to stress. If he can successfully adapt to the stress, or if the stress diminishes or disappears, he returns to normal. But if the stress continues, he eventually reaches the *exhaustion stage,* during which he can no longer resist the effects of stress. In this final stage, physical or emotional disorders may develop; in extreme cases, the person may die.

How much stress a person can handle before reaching the exhaustion stage varies among individuals. Factors affecting a person's ability to cope with stress include his perception of the stressor, intelligence, health, family traits, family diseases, genetic predisposition, environment, and social influences. (See *Identifying stages of the general adaptation syndrome, pages 6 and 7.)*

*Lazarus's theory.* Lazarus also believes that the stress response occurs in three stages, but he views each stage as a conscious evaluation of the stimulus—not as an automatic reaction. In the first stage, the person determines whether the stimulus is irrelevant or stressful; if it's stressful, he decides whether it poses a threat or a challenge. In the second stage, the person chooses his coping strategies. In the third stage, he reevaluates the situation and modifies his strategies as needed.

*Holmes and Rahe's theory.* This theory suggests that all life events—whether positive, such as marriage or a vacation, or negative, such as divorce—cause stress. Thus, the theory focuses not on a single stressor but on the cumulative effects of several stressors over a short period.

Holmes and Rahe have created a social readjustment scale that ranks life events according to how much stress they cause. Of course, the actual amount of stress caused by a particular event will differ for each person. But you can use the scale as a guide to identifying a patient's major stressors and determining the degree of his stress. (See *Social readjustment rating scale,* page 8.)

*General systems theory.* The general systems theory—which sees a person as part of an interrelated system of mind, body, and environment—takes a holistic view of the stress response. The theory recognizes that both internal and external stimuli affect a person's health. Internally, such stimuli as chemical changes or an emotional reaction can have an effect. Externally, such stimuli as the family, the community, and physical surroundings all have an impact. According to this theory, all parts interact, affecting the whole.

***Intrapsychic theory.*** Unlike the general systems theory, Freud's intrapsychic theory focuses only on the psyche. According to this theory, the mind is divided into three basic elements: the id, the ego, and the superego. The *id,* driven by biological needs, compels a person to seek immediate release from any tension, usually with inappropriate behavior. The id might drive a person to walk out of an important meeting in search of food when he's hungry, for instance. The *superego* opposes the id, seeking to suppress all id-driven impulses with internalized morals and values. The *ego* mediates between the two, controlling the id by recognizing and acting according to the rules and limitations of the real world and preventing the superego from imposing excessively strict limitations on behavior. The ego also initiates the defense mechanisms that protect a person from stress.

When these three elements are in balance, a person can function effectively. But severe stress can upset this balance, causing psychosocial problems. Behavioral changes, such as Mrs. Sanchez's withdrawal after her mastectomy, are the outward signs of these inward problems — signs that the ego's defense mechanisms can no longer protect the psyche.

***Cognitive theory.*** Like Freud's intrapsychic theory, the cognitive theory looks within a person rather than at his behavior. But whereas the intrapsychic theory claims that unconscious drives guide a person's behavior and response to stress, the cognitive theory holds that a person can consciously change his behavior, including his reaction to stress. He does this by changing his thinking. The change in behavior then follows,

***Interpersonal theory.*** Instead of looking within the person, the interpersonal theory focuses only on a person's behavior. According to this theory, personality emerges in a person's interactions with others. He relates to people in ways that will bring about physical satisfaction (enough food, rest, physical contact, and sexual fulfillment) and social and emotional security. Stress results when a relationship no longer helps the person meet these needs and instead causes painful emotions. The interpersonal and cognitive theories serve as the bases for most psychosocial nursing theories.

## Coping with stress

All these theories agree on one basic point: When a person experiences stress, he tries to alleviate it. To protect himself from serious discomfort, he uses both unconscious defense mechanisms and conscious, learned responses. Both help him cope when he encounters a stressor, allowing him to regulate his emotional response and take action to change the situation.

### *Coping strategies*

A person under stress has four types of coping strategies he can use. He can change his environment by removing the stressor; for example, a patient might ask you to pull the curtain around his bed to gain a little more privacy. If a person can't change the environment, he may develop ways of dealing with the stressor. For instance, he may learn problem-solving or assertiveness techniques. He can also try to pre-

*(Text continues on page 9.)*

CHECKLIST

# Identifying stages of the general adaptation syndrome

A distinctive set of responses occurs during each of the three stages of the general adaptation syndrome. Use this checklist to help determine which stage your patient is experiencing.

**Alarm stage**
In this stage, stress triggers both sympathetic and parasympathetic responses.

*Sympathetic responses*
☐ Anorexia, constipation, and flatulence
☐ Bronchodilation
☐ Decreased serum chloride
☐ Decreased urine output
☐ Hyperglycemia from glucose buildup
☐ Increased adrenal secretion
☐ Increased blood clotting
☐ Increased blood pressure
☐ Increased body temperature
☐ Increased cardiac contractility, heart rate, and cardiac output
☐ Increased gastric acid secretion
☐ Increased metabolic rate
☐ Increased respiratory rate
☐ Increased serum potassium, glucose, and lactate levels
☐ Inhibited micturition
☐ Mild dehydration
☐ Muscle tension
☐ Peripheral vasoconstriction
☐ Perspiration
☐ Protein catabolism from conversion of protein to glucose
☐ Pupil dilation
☐ Reduced intestinal motility
☐ Short-term increased resistance to inflammation and infection
☐ Sodium and water retention

*Parasympathetic responses*
☐ Bronchoconstriction
☐ Constricted, fixed pupils, leading to blurred vision
☐ Decreased cardiac contractility, heart rate, and cardiac output
☐ Decreased cognition

☐ Dyspnea
☐ Hyperventilation, leading to tremors and dizziness
☐ Hypoglycemia from depleted glycogen stores
☐ Increased gastrointestinal motility, possibly leading to diarrhea
☐ Involuntary or frequent urination
☐ Peripheral flushing
☐ Relaxed muscle tone
☐ Syncope

**Resistance stage**
In this stage, stress causes emotional, cognitive, and physiologic responses.

*Emotional responses*
☐ Aggressive behavior
☐ Alcohol and drug addiction
☐ Anger
☐ Criticism of others
☐ Crying
☐ Depression
☐ Emotional instability
☐ Feelings of helplessness
☐ Feelings of worthlessness
☐ Free-floating anxiety
☐ High-pitched voice
☐ Impatience
☐ Impulsive behavior
☐ Inability to love
☐ Inappropriate laughter
☐ Increased smoking
☐ Increased use of medications
☐ Irritability
☐ Low self-esteem
☐ Negative self-concept
☐ Neurotic behavior
☐ Overreaction to events
☐ Preoccupation with past events
☐ Psychosis
☐ Regressive behavior
☐ Strained relations with others
☐ Stuttering

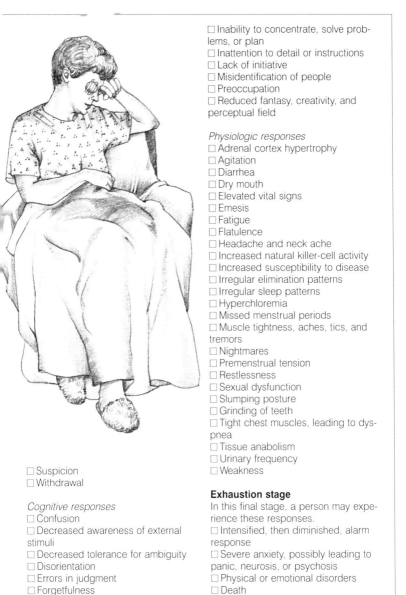

☐ Inability to concentrate, solve problems, or plan
☐ Inattention to detail or instructions
☐ Lack of initiative
☐ Misidentification of people
☐ Preoccupation
☐ Reduced fantasy, creativity, and perceptual field

*Physiologic responses*
☐ Adrenal cortex hypertrophy
☐ Agitation
☐ Diarrhea
☐ Dry mouth
☐ Elevated vital signs
☐ Emesis
☐ Fatigue
☐ Flatulence
☐ Headache and neck ache
☐ Increased natural killer-cell activity
☐ Increased susceptibility to disease
☐ Irregular elimination patterns
☐ Irregular sleep patterns
☐ Hyperchloremia
☐ Missed menstrual periods
☐ Muscle tightness, aches, tics, and tremors
☐ Nightmares
☐ Premenstrual tension
☐ Restlessness
☐ Sexual dysfunction
☐ Slumping posture
☐ Grinding of teeth
☐ Tight chest muscles, leading to dyspnea
☐ Tissue anabolism
☐ Urinary frequency
☐ Weakness

☐ Suspicion
☐ Withdrawal

*Cognitive responses*
☐ Confusion
☐ Decreased awareness of external stimuli
☐ Decreased tolerance for ambiguity
☐ Disorientation
☐ Errors in judgment
☐ Forgetfulness

**Exhaustion stage**
In this final stage, a person may experience these responses.
☐ Intensified, then diminished, alarm response
☐ Severe anxiety, possibly leading to panic, neurosis, or psychosis
☐ Physical or emotional disorders
☐ Death

## Social readjustment rating scale

According to Holmes and Rahe, every event produces a certain amount of stress. Major life changes, such as the death of a family member, cause the most stress, but even seemingly minor events, such as a change in the number of family get-togethers, can cause some stress.

The rating scale below assigns a value to 43 life events. Any combination of events that pushes a patient's total score above 150 can lead to a crisis. A score above 300 signals the possibility of a major life crisis.

(Note that the dollar amounts reflect the cost of living in 1967, when the rating scale was developed.)

| LIFE EVENT | STRESS VALUE | LIFE EVENT | STRESS VALUE |
|---|---|---|---|
| Death of a spouse | 100 | Son or daughter leaving home | 29 |
| Divorce | 73 | Trouble with in-laws | 29 |
| Marital separation | 65 | Outstanding personal achievement | 28 |
| Jail term | 63 | Spouse begins or stops work | 26 |
| Death of a close family member | 63 | Beginning or end of school | 26 |
| Personal injury or illness | 53 | Change in living conditions | 25 |
| Marriage | 50 | Change in personal habits | 24 |
| Fired from job | 47 | Trouble with boss | 23 |
| Marital reconciliation | 45 | Change in work hours or conditions | 20 |
| Retirement | 45 | Change in residence | 20 |
| Change in health of a family member | 44 | Change in schools | 20 |
| Pregnancy | 40 | Change in recreation | 19 |
| Sexual difficulties | 39 | Change in church activities | 19 |
| New family member | 39 | Change in social activities | 18 |
| Business readjustment | 39 | Mortgage or loan less than $10,000 | 17 |
| Change in financial status | 38 | Change in sleeping habits | 16 |
| Death of close friend | 37 | Change in number of family get-togethers | 15 |
| Change to different type of work | 36 | Change in eating habits | 15 |
| Change in number of arguments with spouse | 35 | Vacation | 13 |
| Mortgage over $10,000 | 31 | Christmas | 12 |
| Foreclosure on mortgage or loan | 30 | Minor violations of the law | 11 |
| Change in responsibilities at work | 29 | | |

vent neutral stimuli associated with stressors from turning into stressors themselves. And he can look for ways to divert his attention from the stressor, such as watching television.

The effectiveness of a particular coping strategy will depend on how and when a patient uses it. In some cases, a strategy that's been successful may stop working. When this occurs, help your patient to analyze his problem and adopt appropriate coping strategies.

# Understanding a psychosocial crisis

If a patient's coping strategies fail completely, he may reach a crisis — a state of emotional disequilibrium that he can't correct. A crisis may be either developmental or situational. *Developmental crises* stem from transitional changes that occur throughout life. Crises brought on by marriage, midlife changes, and retirement fall into this category. *Situational crises* occur in response to an unexpected event, such as an illness. (See *How a crisis develops*, page 10.)

Both types of crises have two major characteristics. First, they're self-limiting, usually lasting no more than 6 weeks. Second, they have far-reaching effects. A patient in crisis will adversely affect not only his family but also his entire health care team. He may, for instance, become agitated, resistant, and combative, thereby disrupting the routine of the hospital unit.

A crisis that continues unabated can lead the patient to long-term physical or mental disability, psy-chosis, and even suicide. But a crisis can also open up possibilities for growth. A patient in crisis may be more willing to accept help, especially when he recognizes that his current coping mechanisms won't work. You can then intervene to help him and his family solve the immediate problem that triggered the crisis. And the patient and his family can use new coping skills to deal with the stress that may arise in other situations.

## Phases of a crisis
Different theorists have divided a crisis into distinct phases. By understanding the following theories, you can identify the phase of a patient's crisis and plan the appropriate interventions.

***Caplan's theory.*** Caplan suggests that a person tries his usual problem-solving skills in the initial phase of a crisis. If these fail, his stress increases, leading him to try more extreme coping mechanisms. These may allow him to resolve the problem or redefine it into a problem he can manage. Or these coping mechanisms may allow him to resign himself to the problem or to avoid it. If all his coping mechanisms fail him, major disorganization occurs, leading to mental or physical disorders.

***Tyhurst's theory.*** Tyhurst studied responses to crises in major disasters and identified three phases: the period of impact, the recoil phase, and the posttraumatic period. These phases also apply to other crises, such as those triggered by illness and hospitalization.

The period of impact, of course, refers to the onset of the crisis. During the recoil phase, a person begins to examine how to cope with the crisis. And during the posttraumatic

## How a crisis develops

When a person encounters a stressor that upsets his emotional equilibrium, he follows one of the two paths shown below. If he has adequate coping mechanisms and receives sufficient support, he can resolve the problem before it develops into a crisis. But if the disequilibrium continues unchecked, a crisis results.

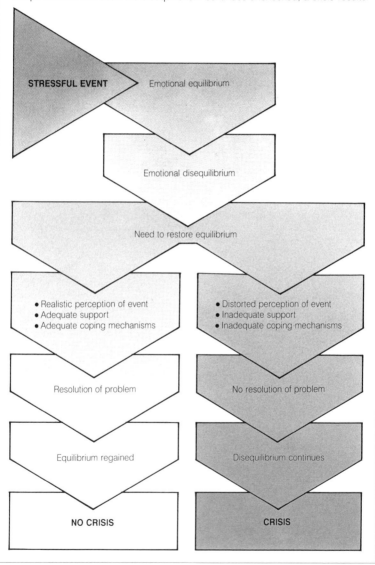

STRESSFUL EVENT › Emotional equilibrium

Emotional disequilibrium

Need to restore equilibrium

• Realistic perception of event
• Adequate support
• Adequate coping mechanisms

• Distorted perception of event
• Inadequate support
• Inadequate coping mechanisms

Resolution of problem

No resolution of problem

Equilibrium regained

Disequilibrium continues

**NO CRISIS**

**CRISIS**

period, he begins to recover from the crisis and function normally again.

**Infante's theory.** Infante also sees crises as occurring in three phases. In the precrisis phase, you can teach your patient coping skills to help him prevent the crisis. During the crisis (the second phase), you can help the patient set priorities, develop attainable goals, and take steps to reach those goals. You may find yourself assessing and intervening simultaneously in this phase to help your patient through the crisis as quickly as possible. In the postcrisis phase, you'll help your patient begin to function normally again.

# Nursing process

To help your patient cope with a psychosocial problem or a full-blown psychosocial crisis, follow the steps of the nursing process — assessment, planning, intervention, and evaluation. The guidelines below can help you use this process most effectively.

## Assessment
Many stressors can trigger a psychosocial crisis, including hospitalization itself. So be alert for signs of a crisis in all your patients. Also, assess a patient for signs of a psychosocial crisis if he experiences any of the following:
• sudden physical illness
• chronic illness
• loss of a body part or a loss of function
• a change in his family (such as a death) during his illness
• the need to change his life-style because of his illness.

Some disorders, such as a myocardial infarction, are more likely to trigger a psychosocial crisis. So you'll need to watch patients with these disorders more closely. A patient with a history of mental illness is also more likely to experience a crisis.

You'll find that assessing some patients is particularly difficult. An aggressive patient or a substance abuser, for instance, may make you feel anxious and frustrated. In such cases, you need to focus on the patient and not be distracted by your reaction. Only by performing an objective assessment of his behavior can you identify his problems. (See *Formulating nursing diagnoses for psychosocial problems,* pages 12 and 13.)

***Assessing coping strategies.*** Find out how the patient perceives the stressful situation and his ability to cope with it. Ask about his usual coping strategies and how they've worked in the past, and look at how well he has coped with previous illnesses.

Do you think the patient is coping effectively? Do his coping strategies seem to help him reach an appropriate outcome? Are his strategies excessive or maladaptive? For instance, is he using an extreme strategy, such as refusing all medications? If so, your assessment may reveal that he doesn't accept his illness.

Based on your assessment of the patient's coping strategies, determine his teaching needs. Does he seem ready to accept change? How important is good health to him? Is he willing to work to regain it? Also make sure he can understand what you intend to teach. If he's not ready or willing to change, he won't respond to your attempts to teach

CHECKLIST

# Formulating nursing diagnoses for psychosocial problems

After observing your patient's behavior, you'll formulate nursing diagnoses to help him resolve his psychosocial problem. The list below contains possible nursing diagnoses of the North American Nursing Diagnosis Association (NANDA) arranged by human response patterns.

**Communicating: A human response pattern involving sending messages**
☐ Impaired verbal communication

**Relating: A human response pattern involving establishing bonds**
☐ Impaired social interaction
☐ Social isolation
☐ Altered role performance
☐ Altered parenting
☐ High risk for altered parenting
☐ Sexual dysfunction
☐ Parental role conflict
☐ Altered family processes
☐ Altered sexuality patterns

**Valuing: A human response pattern involving the assigning of relative worth**
☐ Spiritual distress

**Choosing: A human response pattern involving the selection of alternatives**
☐ Ineffective individual coping
☐ Impaired adjustment
☐ Defensive coping
☐ Ineffective denial
☐ Ineffective family coping: Disabling
☐ Ineffective family coping: Compromised
☐ Family coping: Potential for growth

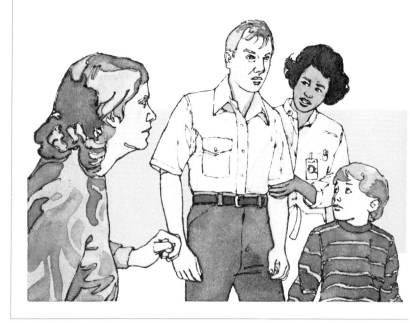

☐ Noncompliance
☐ Decisional conflict
☐ Health-seeking behaviors

**Moving: A human response pattern involving activity**
☐ Sleep pattern disturbance
☐ Diversional activity deficit
☐ Impaired home maintenance management
☐ Self-care deficit
☐ Altered growth and development

**Perceiving: A human response pattern involving the reception of information**
☐ Body image disturbance
☐ Self-esteem disturbance
☐ Chronic low self-esteem
☐ Situational low self-esteem
☐ Personal identity disturbance
☐ Sensory and perceptual alterations
☐ Unilateral neglect
☐ Hopelessness
☐ Powerlessness

**Knowing: A human response pattern involving the meaning associated with information**
☐ Knowledge deficit
☐ Altered thought processes

**Feeling: A human response pattern involving the subjective awareness of information**
☐ Pain
☐ Chronic pain
☐ Anticipatory grieving
☐ High risk for violence: Self-directed or directed at others
☐ Post-trauma response
☐ Rape-trauma syndrome: Compound reaction
☐ Rape-trauma syndrome: Silent reaction
☐ Anxiety
☐ Fear

him more effective coping techniques.

## Planning
Next, work with the patient to set goals he should reach and decide on the interventions that will help him. Listen closely to him to understand his priorities. Remember that they may not be the same as your priorities for him.

Make sure you recognize time limitations. Plan short-term goals that the patient can reach during his hospitalization.

Also consider the patient's capabilities and set achievable goals. Doing so will help you and the patient avoid frustration and a sense of failure.

## Intervention
To help your patient reach his goals, you may use such interventions as therapeutic communication, environmental manipulation, and drug therapy, as ordered. Exactly which interventions you use will depend on the patient and his particular problem. For instance, with a patient suffering severe anxiety, you might try to establish a quiet, soothing environment.

You'll also teach the patient and his family new coping techniques. When you begin, make sure you don't overload the patient with too much information all at once. You may end up increasing his anxiety. And the more anxious he feels, the less he'll learn.

## Evaluation
As you intervene, periodically evaluate the patient's progress. Don't feel disappointed if he's not moving as quickly as you'd hoped he would. Psychosocial changes often occur slowly. Instead, look for signs of progress — no matter how small —

and pass on these results to your patient. When he does meet a goal, decide with him which goal will become his next priority. If he only partially meets a goal, work on developing more effective interventions.

If the patient doesn't meet a goal that you've set, try to determine what went wrong. Do you need to change your interventions? Should you modify the goal? If necessary, you should revise your plan of care. In some cases, you may need to consult a psychiatric clinical nurse specialist or a psychiatrist to develop realistic goals and effective interventions.

# Legal issues

Besides giving your patient the best possible care, you have legal and ethical responsibilities to protect his rights and help him maintain his autonomy. As you know, the American Hospital Association, several professional organizations, and state governments have established bills of rights for patients. Though these bills differ somewhat, they all guarantee certain basic rights. Some patients — such as substance abusers and patients with acquired immunodeficiency syndrome (AIDS) — also have been afforded special guarantees of privacy and confidentiality. (See *Knowing your patient's rights*.)

Protecting these rights can become more challenging when your patient is experiencing a psychosocial crisis. If a patient has completely withdrawn, for example, how can you protect his right to participate in his treatment plan? Is an extremely anxious patient really able to give informed consent? Does a violent patient who may harm himself or others have the right to refuse treatment?

These are some of the thorny questions that can arise when you care for a patient in psychosocial crisis. The discussion that follows centers on two common and crucial issues — informed consent and the use of restraints.

## Informed consent
Informed consent is an agreement by the patient (or someone authorized to act for him) to allow medical or surgical treatment. Such consent protects the patient's autonomy and his right to participate in his treatment. Before he can give his consent, however, he must receive enough information to make a rational decision.

If a patient doesn't give his consent, anyone who performs a procedure or even touches him could be accused of battery. However, if failing to perform the procedure could result in serious harm or death — for instance, if a violent patient must be sedated before he injures himself or someone else — you or the doctor may proceed without consent. If such a situation occurs, make sure you carefully document all circumstances surrounding the incident.

### Who can give informed consent?
Sometimes a patient isn't capable of giving informed consent. In such a situation, someone else — usually a family member — must speak for the patient. In most cases, a minor can give informed consent only if he also has the consent of a parent or guardian. To perform a procedure on a legally incompetent patient, a doctor needs the consent of a guardian or conservator. For an emotionally distressed or mentally ill patient who's considered incapable

of giving consent, the next of kin can usually give consent. If that's not possible, the doctor may need to seek consent from the courts.

***Question of competence.*** To be considered competent enough to decide on medical treatment and give informed consent, a patient must demonstrate reasonable judgment and rational decision making. If he doesn't, he may need a psychiatric evaluation to assess his legal competence. If the psychiatrist can't reach a conclusion about the patient's competence, the courts may have to decide.

Because you spend so much time caring for the patient, you may be the first to notice that he's not making sound judgments. If this happens, document your findings and report them to the doctor. But never simply assume that a patient who's emotionally disturbed or mentally ill is necessarily incompetent. (See *Assessing competence,* page 16.)

***The nurse's role.*** The task of actually explaining the procedure to the patient and obtaining informed consent falls to the person who will perform the procedure — usually the doctor. Your role consists of acting as the patient's advocate and teacher as he considers his decision. You may also witness his signature on the informed consent form.

Remember, though, your responsibility doesn't end when the patient signs the consent form. You should evaluate whether he understands what the doctor has told him and decide if he needs further teaching. You'll need to take extra care when evaluating a patient in psychosocial crisis. An extremely anxious patient may be too agitated to understand what the doctor has told him. Or an abuse victim may identify the doctor

## Knowing your patient's rights

A hospitalized patient has the right to:
☐ receive care in the least restrictive setting
☐ receive appropriate treatment and considerate care
☐ receive complete information about his illness and planned treatment
☐ participate in planning his treatment
☐ know who's involved in his treatment
☐ receive continuous care and appropriate discharge planning
☐ have access to his clinical record, according to hospital guidelines
☐ keep his belongings
☐ have his privacy maintained
☐ have his confidentiality protected
☐ have his civil rights honored
☐ refuse treatment
☐ leave the hospital.

with her abuser and be too frightened to listen to his explanation.

If you think a patient hasn't fully understood what he was told, notify the doctor so that he can take steps to rectify the problem. Otherwise, the consent isn't valid. Keep in mind also that a patient can withdraw his consent at any time.

## Using restraints

At times, a patient in crisis may pose a threat to himself or others. When this happens, you may need to use restraints without his permission.

If you're protecting the patient from falling or pulling out tubes, soft restraints may suffice. Only use locked leather restraints when other methods, such as talking with the patient, changing the environment, and administering medication, have failed to control his violence. And never allow restraints to be used as

## Assessing competence

When you're assessing a patient's competence, consider more than his apparent ability to make a decision about his treatment. After all, a distressed patient may reach a valid conclusion that is based on the wrong reasons — or on no reason at all.

So consider the patient's decisions in other areas of his life, too. For instance, have his recent judgments or decisions seriously disrupted his life? If so, the patient may not be competent despite his treatment decision.

a punishment for unacceptable behavior. If you must use leather restraints, make sure you're familiar with your hospital's policies on their use. These policies reflect federal, state, and local mental health standards.

## Documentation

When you care for a patient experiencing a psychosocial crisis, you'll need to document carefully. Of course, your documentation should always meet the standards spelled out in your hospital's policies. Typically, these standards will be based on criteria established by such organizations as the American Nurses' Association and the Joint Commission on Accreditation of Healthcare Organizations. But when your patient is experiencing a psychosocial crisis, you need to exercise caution.

For instance, when you write progress notes describing a psychosocial problem, be sure you record the patient's behavior patterns. Does the patient always cry after his brother visits? Does he yell only at male staff members? Record such

behaviors and the patient's statements in his own words. Also note the sometimes subtle responses to your interventions. Does the patient seem slightly more at ease after discussing his hostile feelings with you? Be sure to note the time and date for all entries. That way, the interval between the onset of the problem and your intervention and the one between your intervention and the patient's response will be clear to anyone reading your notes.

Finally, if you need to deny one of your patient's rights for therapeutic reasons, document the incident carefully. For example, if you take a belt from a patient who has tried to commit suicide, note exactly what you did and why.

## Suggested readings

Aguilera, D. *Crisis Intervention: Theory and Methodology,* 6th ed. St. Louis: C.V. Mosby Co., 1989.

Backman, M. *The Psychology of the Physically Ill Patient: A Clinician's Guide.* New York: Plenum Pubs., 1989.

Barry, P.D. *Psychosocial Nursing Assessment and Intervention,* 2nd ed. Philadelphia: J.B. Lippincott Co., 1989.

Benner, M.P. *Mental Health and Psychiatric Nursing.* Springhouse, Pa.: Springhouse Corp., 1988.

Burgess, A., ed. *Psychiatric Nursing in the Hospital and the Community,* 5th ed. Norwalk, Conn.: Appleton & Lange, 1990.

Caplan, G. *Principles of Preventive Psychiatry.* New York: Basic Books, 1964.

*Diagnostic and Statistical Manual of Mental Disorders,* 3rd ed., revised. Washington, D.C.: American Psychiatric Association, 1987.

Haber, J., et al. *Comprehensive Psychiatric Nursing,* 3rd ed. New York: McGraw-Hill Book Co., 1987.

Holmes, T.H., and Rahe, R.H. ''The Social Readjustment Rating Scale,'' *Journal of*

*Psychosomatic Research* 11(8): 213-17, 1967.

nfante, M.S. *Crisis Theory: A Framework for Nursing Practice.* Reston, Va.: Reston Publishing Co., 1982.

Iohnson, J., and Lauver, D. "Alternative Explanations of Coping with Stressful Experiences Associated with Physical Illness," *Advances in Nursing Science* 11(2):39-52, January 1989.

Lazarus, R. *Psychosocial Stress and the Coping Process.* New York: McGraw-Hill Book Co., 1966.

Murray, R.B., and Huelskoetter, M.M. *Psychiatric-Mental Health Nursing: Giving Emotional Care,* 3rd ed. Norwalk, Conn.: Appleton & Lange, 1991.

Iorris, J., et al. *Mental Health-Psychiatric Nursing: A Continuum of Care.* New York: John Wiley & Sons, 1987.

*Psychiatric Problems.* NurseReview Series. Springhouse, Pa.: Springhouse Corp., 1991.

Rawlins, R.P., and Heacock, P.E. *Clinical Manual of Psychiatric Nursing.* St. Louis: C.V. Mosby Co., 1988.

Stuart, G.W., and Sundeen, S.J. *Principles and Practice of Psychiatric Nursing,* 4th ed. St. Louis: Mosby-Year Book, Inc., 1991.

Tache, J., and Selye, H. "On Stress and Coping Mechanisms," *Issues in Mental Health Nursing* 7(1/4):3-24, 1985.

Taylor, C.M. *Mereness' Essentials of Psychiatric Nursing,* 13th ed. St. Louis: Mosby-Year Book, Inc., 1990.

Wilson, H.S., and Kneisl, C.R. *Psychiatric Nursing,* 3rd ed. Menlo Park, Calif.: Addison-Wesley Publishing Co., 1988.

# 2

# ASSESSMENT

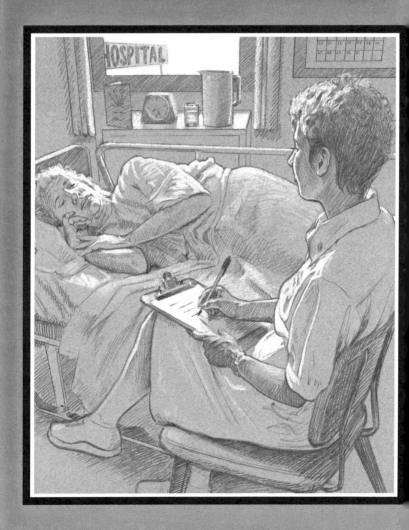

Most patients hospitalized for a physical problem will also have certain psychosocial problems. A patient may, for instance, be anxious about his health or his family's ability to manage while he's hospitalized. Or a patient may be deeply disturbed by a diagnosis he has just received.

Your first inkling of such a problem will probably come when you, another nurse, or a family member notices the patient behaving uncharacteristically. When you get such a hint of a psychosocial problem, you need to assess the patient to determine the cause. Only then can you identify his needs and intervene appropriately.

## Patient responses

Exactly how a particular patient responds to his illness or hospitalization will depend on his past experiences and his mental and emotional status. Keep in mind that a patient's response won't always accurately reflect the seriousness of his illness.

Normal responses to illness range from acceptance to denial. A patient may withdraw or become anxious, depressed, or angry. As he tries to cope with his illness, he may not recognize that he's experiencing emotional or behavioral changes. This doesn't mean that he has a mental illness or an emotional disorder. It just means he needs your help to discover the cause of his problem and to improve his coping skills.

Of course, you may encounter a patient who *does* have a mental illness or an emotional disorder. In some cases, the physical illness may exacerbate a mental or emotional problem that's usually under control. And because of the mental or emotional problem, the patient may be unable to communicate or cope effectively. In such cases, you may need to consult a psychiatric clinical nurse specialist or a psychiatrist to complete the assessment.

# Effective communication

To assess a patient's psychosocial problem, you'll need to conduct an effective interview. That means you must establish a therapeutic relationship based on trust. With your words and actions, let the patient know that his thoughts and behavior are important to you. This promotes trust and helps relieve his anxiety. It also gives you an empathetic understanding of his feelings and needs, which helps you intervene effectively. (See *Establishing a therapeutic relationship,* page 20.)

## Understanding the patient

An ongoing process, communication includes sending and receiving messages and evaluating their meanings. It doesn't, of course, depend entirely on the spoken word. Even when a person tries not to communicate, eye contact, body posture, and the absence of speech send a message. Other nonverbal communicators include facial expression, gestures, clothing, body movements, affect, tone of voice, and voice volume, quality, and pitch.

To communicate effectively during your assessment interview, you must be aware of all these facets of communication. You can also help ensure effective communication by using certain techniques, such as informing, reflecting, confronting, restating, verifying, directing, summarizing, questioning, using silence, and listening. (See *Mastering*

## Establishing a therapeutic relationship

To establish an effective therapeutic relationship with your patient, you need to:
- [ ] actively listen to him and use communication techniques, such as reflection and restatement
- [ ] let him freely express his thoughts, feelings, and experiences
- [ ] be willing to discuss his thoughts, feelings, and experiences
- [ ] evaluate his ability to meet defined goals
- [ ] offer your help
- [ ] encourage him to solve his problems.

*communication techniques.*)

## Communication barriers

Several problems can block effective communication, preventing a successful interview. These include language differences, inappropriate verbal responses, hearing loss, thought disorders, paranoid thinking, hallucinations, delusions, delirium, and dementia.

***Language differences.*** Obviously, you can't communicate effectively if you or your patient uses words the other person doesn't understand. This may occur when a word has more than one meaning — for instance, as a slang term, "bad" actually means good — or when the patient speaks a different language.

If your patient speaks English (or another language you understand), use words appropriate to his educational level, and avoid medical terms he may not understand. Also, keep in mind that intonation, rhythm, speed, pronunciation, and the use of silence will have different meanings in different cultures and countries.

An interpreter can help you communicate with a patient who speaks a language you don't understand. But remember that the presence of a third person may make the patient less willing to share his feelings.

***Inappropriate verbal responses.***
When responding to the patient, choose your words carefully to avoid inhibiting effective communication. For instance, if your patient is expressing his feelings, don't abruptly change the subject or suggest that you're uncomfortable with what he's saying. Be careful not to discount his feelings, offer advice, or tell him how or what he should feel. Also avoid providing false reassurance.

***Hearing loss.*** If you're interviewing a patient with impaired hearing, first check whether he's wearing a hearing aid. If so, is it turned on? If he doesn't have a hearing aid, determine whether he can read lips. If he can, be sure to face him so that he has a direct view of your eyes and mouth. Then speak clearly and slowly, use common words, and make your questions short, simple, and direct. Keep in mind that many hearing-impaired patients don't speak clearly. So be sure you listen carefully to his replies, and ask him to repeat anything you don't understand.

If your patient is elderly, use a low tone of voice. With aging, the ability to hear high-pitched tones deteriorates first. If a patient has a severe impairment, he may have to communicate by writing. Or you may have to collect information from his family or friends.

In some cases, you may need a sign language translator who can also speak, hear, and therefore communicate with you.

CHECKLIST

## Mastering communication techniques

By using the following communication techniques, you can help the patient focus on his feelings, correct misconceptions, and pinpoint ineffective coping mechanisms.

---

☐ *Informing* involves explaining the components or purpose of an activity or procedure. You might, for instance, tell a patient why you're giving him a certain medication.

☐ *Reflecting* involves stating as specifically as possible your understanding of the patient's thoughts and feelings. For example, if the patient says, "I don't need to talk to the doctor about my diagnosis," and acts extremely anxious, you might respond, "You're telling me you're nervous about your diagnosis. Is that right?"

☐ *Confronting* involves describing a contradiction between the patient's words and your perception of his true thoughts or feelings. Tell the patient how his behavior influences your perception, and use a questioning tone of voice to describe the contradiction. Then give him time to respond. For instance, if your patient says he feels calm but seems extremely agitated, you'd need to point out that his actions lead you to believe he's upset, despite his words.

☐ *Restatement* involves summarizing the patient's message in your own words, then allowing him to respond. To a patient who says his treatments "just make me want to scream," you might say, "So what you're saying is that your treatments really upset you."

☐ *Verifying* involves describing your perception of the patient's message in terms similar to the ones he has used. This allows him to confirm or deny that you've understood his message. For instance, if the patient tells you he's angry at himself for getting sick, you'd reply, "You're telling me you think it's your fault you're sick. Is that right?"

☐ *Directing* involves using nonverbal gestures, open-ended questions, and declarative statements to guide the conversation. For instance, when the patient says he hears a voice questioning him, you might look interested and say, "Tell me more about this voice."

☐ *Summarizing* involves reviewing the patient's message in specific terms and clarifying any misconceptions. If a patient scheduled for a painless procedure keeps repeating throughout the session that he's afraid of pain, at some point during or right after your discussion you might say, "It sounds like you're afraid this procedure will hurt. But this is a painless procedure."

☐ *Using open-ended questions* allows the patient to clarify and elaborate on his thoughts and feelings. For instance, you might ask a cancer patient going through radiation therapy how he feels about the therapy.

☐ *Using closed questions* directs the patient toward providing specific information. You might ask your cancer patient specifically if the radiation therapy makes him feel powerless and afraid.

☐ *Using silence* allows the patient to collect his thoughts and reflect on the conversation.

☐ *Listening* allows you to interpret what your patient tells you and to respond appropriately. It also helps you to identify recurring themes in your patient's history and to clarify any statements or issues you don't understand. Above all, conscientious listening lets the patient know you care about him and want to know his problems.

***Thought disorders.*** A patient who's anxious or withdrawn may have illogical, scattered, or incoherent thinking patterns. Because his ideas have no logical connection or focus, his responses may be inappropriate.

When assessing such a patient, ask simple questions about concrete topics and clarify his responses. Let the patient know if you don't understand him, and encourage him to express himself more clearly.

***Paranoid thinking.*** A paranoid patient interprets interpersonal relationships in terms of being persecuted. He's suspicious and mistrustful of others, and acts self-absorbed, rigid, jealous, guarded, and hypersensitive.

When dealing with a paranoid patient, approach him in a nonthreatening way. Avoid touching him because he may misinterpret your touch as an attempt to harm him. Also, keep in mind that he may not mean the things he says.

***Hallucinations.*** Imaginary sensory perceptions with no basis in reality, hallucinations can result from psychiatric disorders, liver failure, drug overdose, or a brain tumor. Five basic types of hallucinations can occur: auditory (the most common), visual, tactile, olfactory, and gustatory.

If your patient is hallucinating, show concern without reinforcing his perceptions. When you give him commands, be as specific as possible. For instance, if he says he's hearing voices, tell him to stop listening to the voices and listen to you instead.

***Delusions.*** A deluded patient accepts false beliefs or ideas and refuses to be swayed by logical reasoning or evidence. Some delusions may be so bizarre that you'll immediately recognize them; others may be difficult to identify until you collect more information.

Don't condemn or agree with a patient's delusional beliefs, and don't dismiss a statement because you think it's delusional. Instead, gently emphasize reality without being argumentative.

***Delirium.*** A delirious patient experiences disorientation, hallucinations, and confusion. Delirium may stem from the use of certain drugs or from a physical problem, such as an infection or a metabolic, cardiovascular, renal, or nervous system disorder.

When interviewing a delirious patient, talk directly to him and ask simple questions. Also, offer frequent reassurance.

***Dementia.*** A usually irreversible deterioration of mental capacity, dementia commonly results from cerebral infarction, Alzheimer's disease, or Parkinson's disease. A demented patient may experience changes in memory and thought patterns, and his language may become distorted or slurred. When interviewing such a patient, minimize distractions, talk simply and concisely, and avoid any statements that could be easily misinterpreted.

# Interviewing the patient

Ideally, the assessment interview should take place in a quiet area where you won't be disturbed. This helps ensure confidentiality and enhances active listening.

If you're meeting the patient for the first time, address him by his surname. Introduce yourself and tell him the purpose of the interview.

After sitting down at a comfortable distance from the patient, give him your undivided attention. Never appear rushed or preoccupied. By creating a relaxed, unhurried atmosphere, you'll make the patient more at ease and assure him that you're willing to listen.

During the interview, be professional but friendly, and maintain good eye contact. Be kind and caring when talking with the patient. Pay close attention not only to what he says, but also to what he's trying to reveal. Use a nonthreatening tone of voice and don't be judgmental.

It may take a while before the patient trusts you enough to offer useful information about his feelings. However, you can still collect important data by observing his behavior.

If your patient becomes acutely anxious, you may have trouble continuing the interview. By dealing with this situation directly, you can help the patient and ensure that the interview is productive. (See *Calming the acutely anxious patient.*)

### Interview methods

How should you conduct your assessment interview? That will depend on you, the patient, and the situation. There isn't one "correct" way to conduct a successful interview. But you should keep the following two general approaches in mind as you decide how to proceed.

*Formal approach.* With this method, you'll use particular assessment tools. Typically, you'll use a general assessment form to assess the biological, social, and psychological needs of your patient. If he has a mental illness, you may use a more extensive psychiatric evaluation form.

You'll also perform either a com-

EMERGENCY INTERVENTION

## Calming the acutely anxious patient

If your patient becomes so anxious or fearful that he can't answer your questions, stop the interview. Then discuss the situation openly with him, using a quiet, reassuring manner. Try to help him identify the cause of his anxiety, and see if you can take steps to minimize or relieve it.

You may also encourage the patient to relax by practicing deep breathing. If he begins to hyperventilate, have him breathe into a paper bag. Contact the doctor of a patient who's having an acute anxiety attack; the doctor may order a tranquilizer.

plete mental status examination or a shortened version of it (see *Methods for assessing mental status quickly,* page 24).

The complete mental status examination explores psychiatric history; general appearance; feeling, mood, and affect; perception, awareness, and level of consciousness; thought processes; memory, intelligence, and language skills; impulse control; judgment; insight; and abstract thinking. For many patients, this examination may not be appropriate.

The shorter versions of the examination take only 5 to 10 minutes. One such shorter version, the mini mental state examination, is an efficient means of measuring cognitive function. This test examines orientation to time and place, registration, attention, calculation, recall, and language and motor skills. If the patient has difficulty writing or reading, you'll need to alter the test accordingly. (See *Conducting the mini mental state examination,* pages 26 and 27.)

With a formal approach, you may

## Methods for assessing mental status quickly

Several rating scales let you assess a patient's mental status quickly. Because these scales are limited in what they measure, they can only give you a general impression of the patient's mental status — not a complete picture. The following chart shows some commonly used rating scales and what they measure.

| RATING SCALE | WHAT'S MEASURED |
|---|---|
| Cognitive assessment scale | General knowledge, mental ability, orientation, psychomotor function |
| Cognitive capacity screening examination | Calculation, language, memory, orientation, recall |
| Extended mental status questionnaire | Higher and lower levels of cognitive function, orientation, remote memory |
| Functional dementia scale | Activities of daily living, affect, orientation |
| Global deterioration scale | Assessment of primary degenerative dementia and stages; includes memory, neurologic, and orientation tests |
| Mental status questionnaire | General knowledge, memory, orientation |
| Mini mental state examination | Attention, calculation, language and motor skills, orientation, recall, registration |
| Nurse's mental status examination | Consciousness, judgment, language, memory, mood, orientation |
| Philadelphia geriatric center examination | Recent memory |
| SET test | Alertness, concentration, problem-solving ability, short-term memory |
| Short portable mental status questionnaire | General knowledge, memory, orientation, subtraction |

also use certain assessment tools to help you measure the severity of a patient's depression. Some examples include Zung's Self-Rating Depression Scale, which can be used as a screening tool, the Beck Depression Inventory, and the Algorithm for Depression.

***Informal approach.*** This method uses a loosely structured conversational format to identify the patient's problem.

Start by stating what you know or perceive to be the problem. For instance, you might say something such as "You look very angry and upset. Tell me what's on your mind." Or: "The nurses think that you seem to be angry about being in the hospital. Can you tell me how you feel?" Working together, you and the patient can investigate ways to solve the problem.

A stressed or mentally ill patient may find it difficult to understand

uestions and develop appropriate
nswers. Keep your questions sim-
le, and ask the patient to repeat
,hat he thinks you have said so
ou're sure he has understood you.

## atient history

)btaining a medical and psychiatric
istory helps establish a baseline for
uture assessments and gives clues
o the underlying or precipitating
ause of the current problem.

When gathering the history, keep
n mind that the patient may not be
. reliable source of information, par-
icularly if he's mentally ill. If possi-
le, verify the data with secondary
ources, such as family members,
riends, and health care personnel.
Also check hospital records from
revious admissions, if possible, and
ompare past problems, behavior,
esponses, interventions, and treat-
nents with the current situation.

When taking the patient's history,
xplore the following information:
hief complaint, present symptoms,
emographic data, socioeconomic
ata, cultural and religious beliefs,
nedications, and physical illnesses.

*hief complaint.* The patient may
ot voice his chief complaint di-
ectly. Instead, you, another nurse,
amily members, or friends may
ote that the patient is having diffi-
ulty coping or is exhibiting unusual
ehavior. If this occurs, you'll need
o determine whether the patient is
aware of the problem. When docu-
nenting the chief complaint, write it
erbatim and enclose it in quotation
narks. For example, you might
vrite something such as: Patient
tates, ''I just haven't felt like I can
andle any more stress lately.''

*resent symptoms.* Find out about
he onset of symptoms, the sus-
ected precipitating cause, the type

and severity of symptoms, and the
patient's response to them. Compare
the symptoms with the patient's
normal functioning.

*Demographic data.* Determine the
patient's age, sex, ethnic origin, primary language, birthplace, religion,
and marital status. Use this information to establish a baseline and vali-
date the patient's record.

*Socioeconomic data.* Patients who
are experiencing economic or personal hardships are more likely to
show symptoms of distress during
an illness. Information about your
patient's educational level, housing
conditions, income, current employment, and family may provide clues
to his current problem.

*Cultural and religious beliefs.* Determine your patient's background and
values, which will affect his response to illness and hospitalization.
As you interview him, remember
that certain questions and behaviors
considered inappropriate in one culture may be sanctioned in another.

*Medications.* Certain drugs can
bring on symptoms of mental illness. Review which medications the
patient is currently taking, including
over-the-counter drugs, and check
for interactions. Also ask about his
use of alcohol and illicit drugs.

If he's taking an antipsychotic,
antidepressant, anxiolytic, or antimanic, does he feel his symptoms
have improved? Is he taking the
medication as prescribed? Is he experiencing any adverse reactions or
allergic responses? If he isn't complying, find out why; adverse reactions may discourage compliance.
(See *Recognizing adverse drug reactions,* page 28.)

*(Text continues on page 29.)*

## Conducting the mini mental state examination

The mini mental state examination quantifies cognitive function and screens for cognitive loss. This examination tests a patient's orientation, registration, attention, calculation, recall, and language and motor skills. To conduct and score the examination, follow these general guidelines:

• Seat the patient in a quiet, well-lighted room.

• Instruct him to listen carefully and then answer each question as accurately as possible.

• Give one point for each correct answer, up to a maximum score of 30.

Usually, a score below 24 indicates cognitive impairment, although this may not be an accurate cutoff for highly or poorly educated patients.

**I. Orientation** (maximum score 10)

Ask, "What is today's date?" Then ask for any information omitted and for other specific information listed. For instance, ask, "Can you also tell me what season it is?" "Can you tell me the name of the hospital?" "What floor are we on?" "What town (or city) are we in?" "What county are we in?" "What state are we in?"

1. Date _____
2. Year _____
3. Month _____
4. Day _____
5. Season _____
6. Hospital _____
7. Floor _____
8. Town/City _____
9. County _____
10. State _____

**II. Registration** (maximum score 3)

Ask the patient if you can test his memory. Then say, "ball," "flag," and "tree" clearly and slowly, taking about 1 second for each. After you've said all three words, ask him to repeat them. This first repetition determines the score (0 to 3), but keep saying the words (up to six trials) until he can repeat all three words. If he doesn't eventually learn all three, recall can't be meaningfully tested.

11. Ball _____
12. Flag _____
13. Tree _____
Number of trials: _____

**III. Attention and calculation** (maximum score 5)

Ask the patient to begin at 100 and count backward by sevens. Stop after five numbers (93, 86, 79, 72, 65). Score one point for each correct number.

14. 93 _____
15. 86 _____
16. 79 _____
17. 72 _____
18. 65 _____

OR

If the patient can't or won't perform this task, ask him to spell the word "world" backward (D,L,R,O,W). The score is one point for each correctly placed letter. For example, DLROW = 5, DLORW = 3. Record how the patient spelled "world" backward: _____

19. Number of correctly placed letters _____

**IV. Recall** (maximum score 3)

Ask the patient to recall the three words you previously asked him to remember (in the registration section).

20. Ball _____
21. Flag _____
22. Tree _____

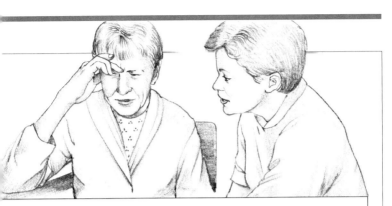

**V. Language and motor skills** (maximum score 9)

• *Naming:* Show the patient a wristwatch and ask, "What is this?" Repeat the question using a pencil. Score one point for each item named correctly.

23. Watch _____
24. Pencil _____

• *Repetition:* Ask the patient to repeat "No ifs, ands, or buts." Score one point for correct repetition.

25. Repetition _____

• *Three-stage command:* Give the patient a piece of blank paper and say, "Take the paper in your right hand, fold it in half, and put it on the floor." Score one point for each action performed correctly.

26. Takes in right hand _____
27. Folds in half _____
28. Puts on floor _____

• *Reading:* On a blank piece of paper, print the sentence "Close your eyes." in letters large enough for the patient to see clearly. Ask him to read it and do what it says. Score one point only if he actually closes his eyes.

29. Closes eyes _____

• *Writing:* Give the patient a blank piece of paper and ask him to write a sentence. It is to be written spontaneously. It must contain a subject and verb and make sense. Correct grammar and punctuation aren't necessary.

30. Writes sentence ___

• *Copying:* On a clean piece of paper, draw intersecting pentagons, with each side about 1", and ask the patient to copy it exactly as it appears. All 10 angles must be present and two must intersect to score one point. Ignore tremor and rotation.

31. Draws pentagons ___

Sample:

*To score the test:* Add the number of correct responses. In section III, include items 14 to 18 or item 19, not both (maximum total score 30).

**Total score** _____

Rate patient's level of consciousness: _____ (a) coma, (b) stupor, (c) drowsy, (d) alert.

Adapted with permission from Folstein, M.F., et al. "Mini-mental State: A Practical Method for Grading the Cognitive State of Patients for the Clinician," *Journal of Psychiatric Research* 12(3):189-98, November 1975.

# Recognizing adverse drug reactions

When assessing a patient, find out which prescription drugs he's taking. If he's taking an antipsychotic, antidepressant, anxiolytic, or antimanic, determine whether he's experiencing any adverse reactions. Common reactions for these drugs are listed below.

**Antipsychotics**  (haloperidol, loxapine, molindone, phenothiazines, thiothixene)
• *Cardiovascular:* arrhythmias, orthostatic hypotension, tachycardia
• *Central nervous system (CNS):* dystonia, extrapyramidal symptoms, neuroleptic malignant syndrome, parkinsonism, seizures, tardive dyskinesia
• *Endocrine:* amenorrhea, changes in libido, galactorrhea, gynecomastia, impotence
• *Eyes, ears, nose, and throat (EENT):* dry mouth, mydriasis, nasal congestion, retinopathy, visual impairment
• *Gastrointestinal (GI):* anorexia, constipation, diarrhea, obstructive jaundice, nausea, vomiting
• *Genitourinary (GU):* urine retention
• *Hematologic:* agranulocytosis, leukocytosis, leukopenia
• *Skin:* dermatitis, photosensitivity

**Antidepressants**  (monoamine oxidase inhibitors, tricyclic antidepressants)
• *Cardiovascular:* arrhythmias, electrocardiogram (ECG) changes, orthostatic hypotension, pedal edema, tachycardia
• *CNS:* delusions, drowsiness, extrapyramidal symptoms, hallucinations, muscle tremors, paresthesia, sedation, tardive dyskinesia
• *Endocrine:* galactorrhea, gynecomastia, hyperglycemia, hypoglycemia
• *EENT:* dry mouth, mydriasis
• *GI:* anorexia, nausea, obstructive jaundice, vomiting
• *GU:* priapism (with trazodone), urine retention
• *Hematologic:* agranulocytosis
• *Skin:* dermatitis

**Anxiolytics**  (benzodiazepines)
• *Cardiovascular:* hypotension, palpitations, syncope, transient ECG changes
• *CNS:* ataxia, confusion, depression, drowsiness
• *Endocrine:* changes in libido
• *EENT:* blurred vision
• *GI:* diarrhea, nausea, vomiting
• *Hematologic:* agranulocytosis, aplastic anemia, neutropenia
• *Skin:* dermatitis

**Antimanics**  (carbamazepine, lithium)
• *Cardiovascular:* arrhythmias, bradycardia, hypotension
• *CNS:* clonic movements, confusion, muscle hyperirritability, slurred speech, tinnitus, tremor
• *Endocrine:* euthyroid goiter, hyperthyroidism
• *EENT:* blurred vision
• *GI:* anorexia, diarrhea, excessive salivation, nausea, vomiting
• *GU:* albuminuria, oliguria, polyuria, decreased creatinine clearance
• *Skin:* alopecia, drying and thinning of hair, itching

***Physical illnesses.*** Find out if the patient has a history of medical disorders that may cause disorientation, distorted thought processes, depression, or other symptoms of mental illness. For instance, does he have a history of renal or hepatic failure, infection, thyroid disease, increased intracranial pressure, or a metabolic disorder?

## General observations
As you interview the patient, you'll also assess his appearance, behavior, mood, thought content, cognitive function, and coping response. A skilled assessment of these factors can reveal how your patient is adapting to his illness.

***Appearance and behavior.*** Closely observe the patient for clues to his emotional state. Specifically, note the following:
• Is his posture erect or slouched? Is his head bowed?
• Is his gait brisk, slow, or shuffling? Does he walk normally?
• Does he look alert or does he stare blankly? Does he appear sad or angry?
• Does he bite his nails, appear restless, or pace? Note his body mechanics.
• Does he make eye contact? Is it constant and intense?
• Does he act cooperative, friendly, hostile, or indifferent to the interviewer?

Also note any speech characteristics that may indicate an alteration in the patient's thought process. These include no response, convoluted or excessively detailed speech, repetitive speech patterns, a flight of ideas, or sudden silence without an obvious reason.

If applicable, observe the patient's clothing and grooming and determine if they're appropriate for

the situation and season.

***Mood.*** Does the patient appear depressed or excited? Is he crying, sweating, breathing heavily, or having tremors?

Ask him how he feels. If he says he feels a certain way—such as anxious or afraid—ask him to describe the feeling. How long has he felt this way? What does he think caused these feelings?

Sometimes a patient's words won't match his facial expression or body language. If he says, "I'm fine, no problems" but looks sad and tearful, he needs your encouragement to talk about his feelings.

***Thought content and cognitive function.*** Evaluate the patient's orientation to time, place, and person, noting any confusion or disorientation. Note any delusions, hallucinations, obsessions, compulsions, fantasies, or daydreams.

Check the patient's attention span and ability to recall events, both past and recent. To check his immediate recall, ask him to repeat a series of five or six numbers or things.

Test the patient's ability to calculate by asking him to add a series of numbers. Test his judgment by asking him what he would do in a particular situation, such as winning the lottery. Be careful not to let your own biases and values cause you to evaluate his answer incorrectly. Finally, test the patient's insight by evaluating how well he understands the significance of his present illness, the anticipated treatment, and the effect the illness may have on his life.

***Coping response.*** Normally, when faced with a stressful situation, a patient will adopt coping or defense mechanisms—behaviors that usually

## Understanding coping mechanisms

Usually operating on an unconscious level, coping mechanisms defend the ego in times of anxiety. The following list defines some commonly used coping mechanisms.

☐ *Denial:* refusing to acknowledge a stressful situation

☐ *Displacement:* transferring an emotion from its original target to another target

☐ *Fantasy:* using nonrational mental activity to escape from daily pressures and responsibilities

☐ *Identification:* unconsciously adopting the personality characteristics, attitudes, values, and behavior of another person

☐ *Projection:* projecting negative feelings onto another individual

☐ *Rationalization:* substituting acceptable reasons for the real reasons motivating behavior

☐ *Reaction formation:* acting in a manner opposite to the way a person feels

☐ *Regression:* returning to the behavior of an earlier, more comfortable time in life

☐ *Repression:* forcing certain thoughts or feelings into the subconscious

☐ *Suppression:* consciously excluding certain thoughts and feelings from the mind

operate on an unconscious level and protect the patient during the stressful situation. They may include denial, regression, displacement, projection, reaction formation, and fantasy. Eventually, the patient has to replace these mechanisms with coping skills that allow him to correct the situation instead of just protecting himself from it. If he doesn't, the coping mechanisms can create problems for both him and the persons interacting with him.

Evaluate your patient for excessive use of these coping mechanisms. (See *Understanding coping mechanisms.*)

# Diagnostic tests

Certain diagnostic tests may provide information about the patient's mental status, particularly if his psychiatric problems result from organic disease. The patient's health history and physical examination will determine which diagnostic tests, if any, should be performed.

### Laboratory tests

The doctor may order laboratory tests — such as urinalysis, hemoglobin, hematocrit, serum electrolyte and serum glucose levels, and liver, kidney, and thyroid function tests — to check for disorders that can cause psychiatric symptoms. He also may order toxicology tests on blood and urine to detect toxic drug levels.

A dexamethasone suppression test, which indirectly measures cortisol hyperactivity, may be used to test for depression. In a patient with depression, cortisol levels will remain elevated or normal for 18 hours after he receives a 1-mg injection of dexamethasone.

### Other tests

To screen for brain abnormalities, a doctor may order an EEG. Abnormal test results may indicate psychotropic drug use.

A computed tomography (CT) scan combines radiologic and computer analysis of tissue density to produce images of intracranial structures. This test can help detect brain contusions or calcifications, cerebral atrophy, hydrocephalus, inammation, space-occupying lesions, and vascular abnormalities.

Magnetic resonance imaging (MRI) takes advantage of certain cell nuclei that magnetically align and then fall out of alignment after a radio frequency transmission. In a process called precession, the MRI scanner records signals from nuclei as they realign; it then translates the signals into detailed pictures of body structures. Compared with conventional X-rays and CT scans, MRI provides superior contrast of soft tissues and a sharper differentiation of normal and abnormal tissues. MRI also provides images of multiple planes, including direct sagittal and coronal views, in regions where bones usually interfere.

Finally, a positron emission tomography scan provides colorimetric information about the brain's metabolic activity by detecting how quickly tissues consume radioactive isotopes.

## Suggested readings

Abraham, I.L., et al. "A Psychogeriatric Nursing Assessment Protocol for Use in Multidisciplinary Practice," *Archives of Psychiatric Nursing* 4(4):242-59, August 1990.

Cohen, G.D. *The Brain in Human Aging.* New York: Springer Publishing Co., 1988.

Corr, D.M., and Corr, C.A. *Nursing Care in an Aging Society.* New York: Springer Publishing Co., 1990.

Cosgray, R. "Understanding Drug Abuse in the Elderly," *Midwife Health Visitor and Community Nurse* 25(6): 222-23, June 1988.

David, A.S. "Insight and Psychosis," *British Journal of Psychiatry* 166:708-808, June 1990.

*Diagnostic and Statistical Manual of Mental Disorders,* 3rd ed., revised. Washington, D.C.: American Psychiatric Association, 1987.

Ebersole, P. *Caring for the Psychogeriatric Client.* New York: Springer Publishing Co., 1989.

Folstein, M.F., et al. "Mini-mental State: A Practical Method for Grading the Cognitive State of Patients for the Clinician," *Journal of Psychiatric Research* 12(3):189-98, November 1975.

Giger, J., and Davidhizar, R.E. *Transcultural Nursing: Assessment and Intervention.* St. Louis: Mosby-Year Book, Inc., 1991.

Green, C. "Have We the Skills?" *Nurse Practitioner* 3(3):26-28, March 1990.

Matzo, M. "Confusion in Older Adults: Assessment and Differential Diagnosis," *Nurse Practitioner* 15(9):32-36, September 1990.

Shea, S. *The Psychiatric Interview: The Art of Understanding.* Philadelphia: W.B. Saunders Co., 1988.

Tillman-Jones, T.K. "How to Work With Elderly Patients on a General Psychiatric Unit," *Journal of Psychosocial Nursing and Mental Health Services* 28(5):27-31, May 1990.

Turnbull, J.M. "Anxiety and Physical Illness in the Elderly," *Journal of Clinical Psychiatry* 50(11, Suppl):40-45, November 1989.

Varcarolis, E.M. *Foundations of Psychiatric Mental Health Nursing.* Philadelphia: W.B. Saunders Co., 1990.

Worley, N.K., and Albanese, N. "Independent Living for the Chronically Mentally Ill," *Journal of Psychosocial Nursing and Mental Health Services* 27(9):18-23, September 1989.

# 3

# BEHAVIORAL PROBLEMS

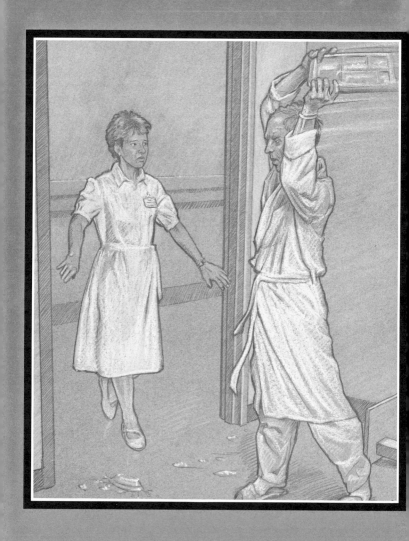

A patient who behaves abnormally isn't necessarily showing signs of a psychiatric disorder. In fact, he may be a normally calm, rational person who's simply responding to the stress of his illness and hospitalization. Or he may have a preexisting behavioral problem that's normally in check but that surfaces when he experiences extreme stress. Or he may have an uncontrolled behavioral problem that's not caused by a psychiatric disorder.

Behavioral problems take many forms, and they have various origins. Physical and emotional stress may trigger feelings of helplessness, insecurity, and loss of control; may threaten the patient's dignity, self-esteem, and sense of well-being; and may cause fear of the unknown and even a fear of death.

But no matter what the nature of a patient's behavioral problem, he needs helpful, understanding care from you. So when caring for a patient with such a problem, remember that his adjustment to his illness and hospitalization will take some time and that he'll require skillful nursing intervention to help him deal more effectively with stress.

**Dealing with your feelings**

Patients with behavioral problems can affect caregivers in different ways. Depending on your patient's behavior, you may experience feelings of rejection, defensiveness, avoidance, impatience, irritation, anger—even hostility. Despite your best efforts to hide your feelings, you may nevertheless convey them to the patient nonverbally (such as by your body language), thus exacerbating his anxiety.

You'll need to accept that reacting to your patient's behavioral problems with uncomfortable or negative feelings is perfectly normal. Once you've recognized that the patient isn't directing his behavior at you personally, but rather at the situation he's in, you can begin to work through your feelings.

When working with a difficult patient, you have to recognize how he makes you feel and explore the reasons behind his behavior. Talking about the situation with a trusted peer, a psychiatrist, or a psychiatric clinical nurse specialist, or discussing it in a staff meeting, may help you. But you should resist the natural temptation to absolve yourself of any responsibility in dealing with a difficult patient. When you're able to work through your own reactions, the patient may sense it and perceive a more accepting, comforting environment. And you may find that he's ready to moderate his abnormal behavior.

This chapter discusses specific behavioral problems commonly seen in hospitalized patients. These include manipulation, noncompliance, aggression, inappropriate sexual behavior, malingering, and obsessive-compulsive and dependent behavior. You'll find a discussion of the characteristics of each problem. Plus, you'll learn key assessment steps, nursing interventions, and evaluation measures for patients with such problems.

# Manipulative patient

Purposeful behavior used by a person to get what he wants, manipulation isn't always a behavioral problem. Positive manipulation uses constructive interpersonal skills to promote successful relationships with others. As a nurse, you use

CHECKLIST

## Are you being manipulated?

Watch for patient behaviors that indicate possible manipulation, including:
- [ ] flattery
- [ ] overfriendliness
- [ ] overtalkativeness
- [ ] feigned compliance
- [ ] helplessness
- [ ] playing staff members against each other
- [ ] tearfulness
- [ ] slowness
- [ ] gift giving
- [ ] negativity
- [ ] threats
- [ ] seductive dressing or body language
- [ ] excessive criticism
- [ ] refusal to participate
- [ ] excessive smiling
- [ ] sarcasm.

positive manipulation everyday to get positive responses from your patients. For example, by complimenting a paraplegic patient on his successful transfer from a bed to a wheelchair, you're using a type of manipulation to promote self-confidence and motivation in the patient.

However, manipulation *is* a behavioral problem when the patient:
- uses it as the primary method to get what he wants
- disregards others' feelings
- treats others disrespectfully or as objects to fulfill his needs.

Maladaptive manipulation commonly develops in childhood, as the child discovers that he can use it to get his parents' attention or fulfill his other needs and desires. The child who effectively uses manipulation in this way usually continues to do so as an adult.

Manipulative behavior typically masks hidden fears, a lack of trust in relationships, and feelings of insecurity. The manipulator doesn't trust others to meet his needs if he communicates them directly. His desire to control these feelings prompts the manipulative behavior in varying degrees.

In the hospital, a manipulative patient has an excessive fear of losing control. Routines, rules, and procedures cause a feeling of powerlessness. Increased anxiety triggers maladaptive manipulation.

### Assessment

During your assessment of the manipulative patient, you should look for characteristic behaviors, including distracting maneuvers, disparaging maneuvers, and aggressive maneuvers. Keep in mind that the patient may use various behaviors simultaneously and may try different behaviors to find out which one works for him. (See *Are you being manipulated?*)

Used to provoke guilt or frustration in caregivers, *distracting maneuvers* include overfriendliness, flattery, excessive talkativeness, feigned compliance, helplessness, tearfulness, dawdling, slowness, and constantly changing the subject of conversation.

Slightly more forceful in nature, *disparaging maneuvers* — reprimands, criticism, complaints — aim to promote feelings of inadequacy in staff members.

*Aggressive maneuvers* are the most obvious type of manipulative behavior. They include making unrealistic demands, questioning each step of a procedure, using coercion, attempting to play staff members off of each other, violating rules and routines, making stipulations or verbal threats, and even acting out aggressively.

Another, more serious aggressive maneuver involves threatening self-destructive behavior, such as self-abuse or suicide. The patient does this in an attempt to provoke discomfort, fear, and self-doubt in caregivers. On the unit, an aggressive manipulator may assume a ''leadership'' role (for example, organizing other patients to oppose a staff member) and can be a major disruptive force.

*Examining your feelings.* A nurse who's personally or professionally insecure is most susceptible to manipulation. But anyone can be a victim. An expert manipulator can readily detect a person's weaknesses and play on them to get what he wants. To deal with such a patient effectively, you have to first explore how his behavior makes you feel. Failure to do so can lead to other problems. For example, if you don't recognize your unresolved feelings of hostility toward a patient, you'll find it more difficult to establish a therapeutic relationship with him, and you may end up avoiding him or punishing him in some way. You may feel frustrated or angry and end up behaving in a manner similar to that of the patient. (See *Nurse-patient manipulation cycle,* page 36.)

## Intervention

Nursing interventions for manipulative behavior are not intended to control the patient, but rather to provide consistent guidelines to help him gain self-control. You can help build the manipulative patient's trust by showing him how to fulfill his needs without using manipulation.

*Setting goals.* For most patients — those who will be in the hospital for only a short stay — you should focus on achieving short-term goals by a certain date. These goals typically include having the patient:
• demonstrate some improvement in his manipulative behavior
• show greater trust in the staff
• demonstrate increased self-esteem
• express thoughts and feelings directly.

*Confronting the patient.* After identifying the patient's manipulative behavior, try to determine why he feels the need to use it. Taking a nonthreatening, nonjudgmental approach, ask him why he acts this way. Tell him how his behavior makes you feel. For example, say to him, ''I feel angry and embarrassed when you belittle me in front of the other patients.'' Then ask him what he's feeling and experiencing when he acts manipulative. This approach can help the patient identify his manipulative behavior and the feelings that generate it. Confront the patient each time you observe manipulative behavior in him, and discuss alternate coping techniques for dealing with the situations or the people that trigger it. For instance, when the patient feels the desire to manipulate, he can state his needs directly instead. Or he can substitute assertive behavior for manipulative behavior.

*Maintaining a calm approach.* Discuss the patient's manipulative behavior calmly and matter-of-factly. Avoid accusing, arguing, or getting involved in power struggles with the patient, which can only exacerbate the problem. Instead, focus on maintaining self-control in order to deal with the situation constructively.

*Setting limits.* Set firm, consistent,

## Nurse-patient manipulation cycle

Failure to resolve conflicts between you and a manipulative patient can trigger a cycle of manipulation and hostility, as shown below.

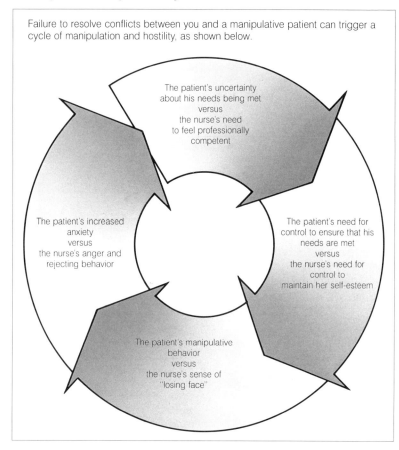

The patient's uncertainty about his needs being met versus the nurse's need to feel professionally competent

The patient's need for control to ensure that his needs are met versus the nurse's need for control to maintain her self-esteem

The patient's manipulative behavior versus the nurse's sense of "losing face"

The patient's increased anxiety versus the nurse's anger and rejecting behavior

reasonable limits on specific behaviors. (See *How to set limits.*) For example, tell the patient that he can't smoke in his room but can smoke in the lounge. Recognize that although the patient may resist such limits outwardly, he really desires them. To help him accept limits, explain that setting limits promotes discipline without the threat of punishment.

*Providing positive feedback.* Pro-

mote direct, open communication. Be honest, forthright, and assertive. Assist the patient in testing alternative behaviors — such as positive communication techniques, assertiveness, and direct confrontation — that help him cope with his problems. When responding to a direct request, make every attempt to meet the patient's needs, so he won't feel he has to resort to indirect manipulation to get what he wants. Give positive feedback when the patient demonstrates honest, open communication and appropriate behavior.

***Ensuring consistent care.*** If possible, work with the patient exclusively long enough to develop a therapeutic, trusting relationship. As this relationship develops, the patient's anxiety should decrease. You'll also become more familiar with his behavior and be better able to support him, set limits more consistently, and evaluate the effectiveness of your interventions.

***Maintaining a safe environment.*** You need to ensure the patient's safety, regardless of how difficult his behavior may make this. Take all of his self-destructive threats seriously, and explore the feelings behind the threats. Keep in mind that a manipulative patient may make threats to test your concern for him. Make sure he knows that you will take all of his threats seriously and that you will report them to the doctor.

### Evaluation
Evaluate the patient's response to interventions by examining goals set and goals achieved. Be prepared for some initial problems; limit setting commonly provokes anger and further manipulation. But once the patient tests the limits and sees that you're enforcing them, you can expect him to feel a sense of security. Give him time to experiment with his new adaptive behaviors. As his trust increases, look for him to use more direct, open communication and to replace manipulative behavior with more appropriate means of getting his needs met.

Keep in mind that a patient who transfers to another floor or is discharged early may not achieve all of

## How to set limits

Follow these guidelines to set limits on your manipulative patient's behavior.
☐ Only set limits on behavior that clearly threatens the patient or others.
☐ Allow the patient some freedom within set limits to give him a sense of control.
☐ Determine realistic and enforceable consequences for nonadherence to limits.
☐ Clearly communicate the limits and consequences to the patient; permit the patient to express his feelings about them.
☐ Ensure that all limits and consequences are specified in the care plan and that all staff members are familiar with them.
☐ Ensure that staff members consistently enforce the limits and implement the consequences when necessary.
☐ Remove limits from the care plan once the patient consistently demonstrates nonmanipulative behavior.

his goals. If this happens, examine your own emotional response and, if you feel the need, share it with other staff members who have worked with the patient. To combat negative feelings, such as anger and frustration, remember that any behavioral change takes time and that even though the patient may not have achieved all of his goals, you've taught him skills that he may find helpful later.

***Requesting a consultation.*** Depending on the circumstances, you may request a consultation at any point in the nursing process. Typically, you'll assess, intervene, and evaluate the patient before consulting with a psychiatrist or psychiatric clinical nurse specialist.

Sometimes, though, a consultation may need to take place earlier. For instance, notify the doctor whenever the manipulative patient expresses threats of any nature. Such a patient may need to be moved to a psychiatric facility to ensure his safety — and that of others. Also, as soon as you identify a behavioral problem, you may want to consult with a psychiatric clinical nurse specialist, who can help evaluate both the patient's and your underlying feelings, set realistic goals, plan appropriate interventions, and help you better deal with your feelings, thus promoting a therapeutic nurse-patient relationship.

# Noncompliant patient

A common behavioral problem in patients, noncompliance is the willful resistance to a prescribed care regimen. Examples of noncompliance include the diabetic patient who won't follow dietary guidelines, the obese hypertensive patient who won't lose weight, and the arthritic patient who won't take his medication.

A patient commonly will offer excuses for noncompliance — for example, insufficient time or money. In most cases, this type of rationalization helps alleviate the anxiety that underlies the patient's noncompliance. For instance, a patient may deny the seriousness of his illness because he's afraid of dying, and his noncompliance may help protect him from the overwhelming anxiety he'd feel if he admitted how ill he actually is.

In other cases, a patient may use noncompliance to gain control over his body and his fate. For example,

a cardiac patient who doesn't take his medication as prescribed may think he still has control of his body. Most chronically ill patients need to test the limits of their control and the validity of the prescribed regimen.

## Assessment
To better understand a patient's noncompliance and plan interventions accordingly, review his history. If the patient is a child, you can begin to assess behavioral impasses by talking to his parents or guardians. Ask them how the child behaves at home. Do they discipline him? How? Find out if they set consistent limits. How well does the child understand his physical problem? How well does he communicate?

If the patient is an adult, ask him how long he's had this illness. What is his understanding of his illness? Find out how it has affected his life. Why does (or doesn't) he view this illness as problematic? Ask if he's been hospitalized before. If so, what were the reasons (physical or mental illness) and how did hospitalization affect him and his family?

As appropriate, explore other related issues, such as alcohol or drug use (or abuse), available support systems, recent traumatic experiences (for example, divorce or death in the family), and the usual coping mechanisms of noncompliance, including denial, rationalization, minimizing the problem, and projecting the problem onto others.

If your patient is elderly, also ask him whether he lives in a special residence for the elderly. Do any physical or mental limitations interfere with his life-style? Does he have adequate support systems? Ask him if any family members live nearby.

After reviewing the patient's history for clues to his behavioral problems, you may need to further explore possible reasons for his noncompliance. (See *Assessing noncompliance.*) Of course, you also need to assess any physical consequences of his noncompliance.

If the patient's resistant behavior directly threatens his life or well-being, make physiologic treatment your first priority.

*Examining your feelings.* To intervene effectively, you need to understand your own feelings about the patient's noncompliance. Common responses to noncompliance include anger, frustration, and impatience. As a nurse, you probably find it very difficult to observe self-destructive behavior without intervening to stop it. For this reason, you may not tolerate noncompliance and may tend to distance yourself from the patient.

### Intervention

As discussed earlier, set priorities for your interventions so that you deal first with any noncompliance-related problems that will harm the patient. For instance, if a diabetic patient constantly eats candy, you'll need to set limits to discourage him and help prevent complications, such as hyperglycemic coma.

*Exploring the patient's feelings.* Encourage the patient to express what he understands about his illness and hospitalization, what he feels is happening to him, and why he's anxious. Using such communication techniques as active listening, clarifying, and reflecting, encourage him to identify and talk about his feelings. Correct any misinformation or misconceptions about the treatment and illness. Strive to develop a ther-

## Assessing noncompliance

To explore why a patient is noncompliant, ask yourself these questions.

**Psychological considerations**
• Does the patient lack important knowledge?
• What are his beliefs and values?
• Is he denying his illness?
• What is his anxiety level?
• What is his personality type?
• Is he motivated to improve his physical status?

**Environmental and social considerations**
• What are the patient's cultural beliefs and values?
• Is his support system effective?
• Does he have problems that can affect health care and self-care—for example, financial difficulties, lack of transportation, or homelessness?

**Treatment considerations**
• Are the patient's expectations of treatment too high or too low?
• Is he physically capable of carrying out the treatment plan?
• How helpful is the treatment?
• What are the benefits versus the adverse effects of the treatment?
• Does the patient understand what will happen if he's not treated?
• How does he think the treatment will improve his physical health?
• Is he pessimistic about his health? Does he believe that the treatment won't help? Why?

**Therapeutic relationship**
• Is the patient being treated with respect by health care providers?
• Is communication effective?
• Is there a power struggle between the patient and health care providers?
• How does the patient view the health care providers? As empathetic and helpful? Or as rigid and controlling?

## Understanding the nurse-patient contract

An oral or written agreement between a nurse and a patient regarding their behavior toward one another, a nurse-patient contract can help promote patient compliance. A written contract, such as the sample presented below, clearly specifies the agreed-upon behaviors and is dated and signed by both the nurse and the patient.

CONTRACT

Date __2/3/92__ and __Doris Rosen, RN__
(nurse's name)
__John Martin__ until __2/8/92__
(patient's name) (date)
agree that from __2/4/92__ (date)
they will do the following.

The patient will: *request assistance and wait for a staff member to arrive before attempting to get out of bed.*

The nurse will: *inform all staff members to answer the patient's request within five minutes and assist patient out of bed.*

__Doris Rosen, RN__
(nurse's signature)

__John Martin__
(patient's signature)

apeutic relationship that promotes understanding, trust, and continuity of care.

***Collaborating with the patient.*** By forming a collaborative relationship with the patient, you can develop joint agreements or contracts that allow him to accept increasing responsibility for his own care. Negotiate what you can do for the patient and what he can do for himself. (See *Understanding the nurse-patient contract.*)

Become familiar with the patient's health care goals, and use them appropriately in planning care. You may need to accept the fact that the patient's goals aren't the same as yours. However, make sure that all goals are realistic and attainable. Discuss with the patient the steps necessary to meet the goals. Try to set easily achieved goals at first; accomplishing them may increase the patient's determination to progress.

***Developing effective coping mechanisms.*** Try to identify the patient's normally effective coping mechanisms, then encourage him to apply those same coping mechanisms to his current problem. As necessary, consult with a psychiatric clinical nurse specialist to develop interventions aimed at encouraging more effective coping strategies.

***Providing support.*** Offer positive feedback when the patient attempts to comply with the care regimen. Encourage family members to express their fears and concerns about the patient's behavior and to learn how to help him. Explain to them that they can best help the patient by encouraging him to perform self-care activities, rather than by providing the care themselves. If necessary, refer the patient and his family to appropriate community resources. For example, if the patient is having difficulty complying with a weight-loss regimen, refer him to Weight Watchers or a similar program.

Discuss the patient's noncompliance problems and your efforts to change his behavior with the home health nurse. This will enable her to provide follow-up care and support for the patient after his discharge.

### Evaluation

Expect a patient who is responding favorably to nursing interventions to accept treatment, to be involved in collaborative efforts to avoid problematic behavior, and to be able to communicate his feelings and identify stressors. He'll also demonstrate adaptive behavior by performing self-care measures.

Keep in mind, however, that if you're with the patient for only a short time, you may not be able to properly evaluate his degree of compliance because you can't observe his behavior after his discharge. The home health nurse or a nurse in another health care setting may have to complete this last step.

*Requesting a consultation.* If the patient's noncompliance persists or worsens despite your interventions, request a consultation with a psychiatrist or psychiatric clinical nurse specialist. This is especially important for a patient who is giving any

indication that he intends to harm himself or others.

If the psychiatrist concludes that the patient's behavioral symptoms result from a physical illness, you can expect his symptoms to abate as his illness becomes resolved. If the patient's behavior results from anxiety, the psychiatrist may prescribe an anxiolytic drug such as diazepam.

The psychiatric clinical nurse specialist can give you additional insight into predisposing factors that cause noncompliance and associated behavioral patterns. She may also help you deal with your own negative feelings so that they don't interfere with your therapeutic relationship with the patient.

# Aggressive patient

Actions performed to gratify the need to excel, achieve, or compete within or separate from the group, aggression can be positive or negative. Positive aggression is aggression that's channeled into an appropriate outlet, such as a competitive sport. Negative aggression includes physical aggression (behavior that results in harm to oneself or another, or destruction of property) and verbal aggression (threats or gestures that evoke fear in another, whether intentionally or not). Aggression generally stems from anger and frustration.

### Assessment

When dealing with a potentially aggressive patient, you need to recognize preaggressive behavior and subsequent stages so that you can intervene quickly and halt the cycle before it escalates into violence.

## Understanding the stages of violent behavior

You need to recognize the stages of violent behavior so that you can intervene at the earliest possible moment and prevent harm to the patient and others. These stages of violent behavior include:

*Increasing anxiety*
The patient exhibits diverse minor changes, such as staring, shaking, indirect eye contact, gritting teeth, tapping hands or feet, and biting nails. Somatic symptoms include sweating and rapid breathing.

*Verbal threats*
The patient starts making threats. For example, he may say, "I'm going to kill you" or "I'm going to get even with both you and my doctor."

*Hyperactivity (major motor changes)*
The patient demonstrates exaggerated behavior. For example, he begins moving around more, yelling, pacing, or slamming doors. He may walk away from you or refuse to talk to you, cooperate with procedures, or eat.

*Physical aggression or violence*
The patient demonstrates violent behavior. He may have a weapon, such as a gun, or he may use available objects as weapons, such as an ashtray or a telephone. He also may use his fists. The object of his aggression may be himself, an object, or another person, such as you, another patient or staff member, or a visitor.

*Exhaustion*
The patient ceases his aggressive behavior and becomes exhausted.

(See *Understanding the stages of violent behavior* for more details.) Look for characteristic behavioral and emotional cues. Behavioral cues can progress from minor motor changes (such as foot tapping and punching the palm of the hand) to verbal threats, major motor changes (such as pacing, hyperactivity, and punching at walls), physical aggression, and exhaustion. Emotional cues include anxiety, hostility, anger, and rage.

When assessing a patient's behavior, be aware of your own emotional response to him. Your feelings of discomfort — anxiety, tension, and vulnerability — may be early signs alerting you to impending violence.

**Reviewing the patient's history.** Exploring the patient's history may reveal a predisposition to aggressive behavior. (See *Risk factors for violence.*) During the interview, ask the patient about any negative behavioral changes associated with drug or alcohol use. Note any history of frequent fights, criminal activity involving violence, or hospitalization that resulted from aggressive or violent behavior. Also note the patient's socioeconomic background. A person in a subculture in which violence is more prevalent will tend to react more violently to stressful situations.

If you sense the possibility of violent behavior, ask the patient questions that won't tend to provoke a negative response. For example, ask him, "Do you feel like hurting yourself or anyone else?" By asking direct questions, you'll encourage him to communicate openly instead of acting out.

**Observing the patient.** Physical findings may also alert you to the possibility of an aggressive response to stress. Look for scars that may suggest injury caused by self-mutilation or fighting.

*Pinpointing the cause.* When a patient behaves aggressively, you must first control the aggression. Then you can explore the possible causes. Check for evidence pointing to physiologic causes of aggressive behavior, such as alcohol or drug intoxication or withdrawal. Assess for hyperreflexia, nystagmus, dilated pupils, slurred speech, tremors, needle tracks, an eroded nasal septum, or other signs of drug use. If appropriate, consult with the doctor about a toxicology screen to confirm alcohol or drug abuse.

Keep in mind that aggression may also accompany various physiologic disorders. These include hypoglycemia, renal failure, chronic obstructive pulmonary disease, cardiac disease, hormonal or endocrine disorders, neurologic damage secondary to injuries, organic brain syndrome in elderly patients, and neurologic disorders, such as brain tumors, rabies, encephalitis, and temporal lobe epilepsy.

Suspect an organic cause in a patient with a sudden onset of aggressive behavior (possibly accompanied by disorientation and hallucinations), a known medical illness, abnormal vital signs, and no history of any psychiatric disorder. Expect to obtain laboratory tests, including a complete blood count, serum electrolyte studies, hepatic and renal studies, arterial blood gas levels, and an electrocardiogram, to help confirm or rule out organic disease.

Be aware that aggressive behavior may be a sign of a psychiatric disorder, such as dementia, schizophrenia, depression (agitated), a personality disorder (borderline or antisocial), or mania. Such behavior

## Risk factors for violence

Be alert for impending violent behavior in a patient with one or more of the following risk factors:
☐ agitation, disorganized behavior, anger
☐ alcohol or drug intoxication
☐ available means of inflicting injury (for example, possession of a weapon)
☐ demographic factors associated with increased prevalence of violence (male, age 15 to 24, low socioeconomic group, low educational level, social instability due to frequent moves, poor or absent family ties); the risk rises as the number of factors increases
☐ expressed threats of violence
☐ history of physical abuse as a child
☐ history of violent behavior
☐ organic, borderline, or antisocial personality disorder
☐ organic brain syndrome
☐ psychosis, especially paranoid delusions or hallucinations
☐ uncooperativeness.

may also result from mental retardation or an attention deficit disorder. Aggressive behavior can signal a conduct disorder in an adolescent or an explosive disorder in an adult.

Expect certain types of patients to be more prone to aggressive behavior. A patient with a personality disorder tends to be emotionally immature and to have a low frustration threshold. He commonly exercises poor judgment, feels he must have his needs met immediately, lacks guilt feelings for any negative results of his behavior, and reacts aggressively toward anyone perceived as causing him frustration.

A patient with paranoid schizophrenia is prone to violence. He may respond to delusions of persecution by retaliating against the presumed source of the harassment, or he may obey command hallucinations that order him to act violently. In some cases, the patient may become so confused that he unintentionally causes violence through purposeless, excited motor activity. For instance, he may throw whatever he has in his hands or tear at his own or another person's clothing. A manic patient may become violent if you ignore or deny his demands.

***Examining your feelings.*** To deal effectively with an aggressive patient, you need to be aware of your own responses to anxiety, anger, and aggression. Just as the aggressive patient goes through a cycle of escalation, you'll go through a cycle that typically begins with feelings of empathy and escalates to anxiety, fear, anger, counter-aggression, and finally frustration. If you don't deal with these feelings, you may respond in a nontherapeutic, unproductive way. For example, you may distance yourself from the patient; react defensively, aggressively, or condescendingly; and even punish the patient. Instead of working toward a common goal, you and the patient become enemies, thus preventing effective problem solving.

## Intervention
Plan your nursing interventions according to the patient's stage within the escalation cycle.

***During the preaggressive stage.*** If you note preaggressive behavior, use therapeutic communication and limit setting to try to prevent an escalation to violence.

*Using therapeutic communication.* By simply talking to the preaggressive patient, you may be able to

help him feel less threatened and more in control, and thus reduce the risk of injury. Keep in mind that in most cases, the patient is terrified of losing control and really wants you to prevent him from becoming violent.

By using therapeutic communication skills, such as open-ended questioning and offering to work on the patient's problem with him, you can help him identify and discuss his fears and frustrations, which may prevent further escalation. Without intervention at this stage, the patient's frustration and anxiety will only increase, making intervention at the next stage more difficult.

Don't distance yourself from a patient who becomes verbally abusive. A common response, distancing yourself places the patient in psychological seclusion, increasing his fear of abandonment and setting the stage for further escalation. Instead, use talk-down techniques to develop a verbal alliance with him.

*Talk-down techniques* let the patient know that you care, that you won't harm him, and that you won't be afraid of losing control of the situation if his preaggressive behavior returns. You can use three proven talk-down techniques.

In *dislocation of expectations,* you disarm a verbally aggressive patient by reacting to verbal threats not defensively, as he expects, but rather in a calm, nonthreatening, confident manner. Once the patient realizes that you aren't intimidated or frightened, he'll recognize that the situation isn't that threatening, and he may calm down.

In another technique, known as *overdosing,* you find something to agree with in what the patient is saying. For instance, if he's complaining about the care he has been given, find something about his complaint that's true and tell him that you agree. He'll recognize that you're interested in helping him find a solution to his problem.

The third technique, *clarifying emotional status,* is based on the fact that a person cannot feel two opposing emotions simultaneously. In this technique, you respond to a patient expressing anger or making verbal threats with a less threatening emotion. For example, say to him, "You sound as though you're feeling a lot of emotional pain." Although the patient may not respond calmly and rationally at first, he should eventually settle down.

*Setting limits.* Recognize that the patient making threats has the ability to carry them out. If you don't, he may interpret your reaction as a challenge. As appropriate, set limits on his behavior. Clearly explain to him that violence is unacceptable and describe the consequences of any violent behavior, such as the use of restraints or seclusion.

**During the aggressive stage.** If the patient becomes aggressive or violent, your interventions include protecting yourself, subduing the patient (using medication or restraints), and treating the patient (using medication).

*Protecting yourself and others.* If the patient becomes violent, take appropriate action at once. If necessary, remove other patients from the area for their own protection. Remain at a safe distance from the patient, and continue using "talkdown" techniques and providing reassurance to help him regain control of himself. If you feel unsafe, you or someone else should call security.

For your own safety, always provide yourself with an escape route

# If your patient has a weapon

If a patient tells you that he has a weapon, or if you see that he has one, follow these guidelines:
- Don't immediately demand that he relinquish the weapon. This may heighten his intense feelings and increase his agitation.
- Notify hospital security.
- If the patient indicates that he wants to relinquish the weapon, don't take it from him. Instead, have him place it on a bedside table or stand.
- If he threatens you with the weapon, calmly state that he's frightening you. Don't attempt to subdue, argue with, or threaten him—this could trigger an assault.

to get away from a violent patient. Never back yourself into a corner or allow the patient to block the doorway. Be prepared to move quickly; a violent patient may attack suddenly. If possible, have pillows available to use as protection. (See *If your patient has a weapon* for information on how to react to an armed, violent patient.)

*Immediate drug therapy.* As ordered, administer an antianxiety agent, a phenothiazine, or a sedative hypnotic medication while other staff members hold the patient down. These drugs may quickly reduce anxiety, agitation, and hyperactivity in some patients, quelling aggressive or violent behavior.

*Applying restraints.* You'll apply mechanical restraints to subdue a patient only as a last resort. But if you need to apply restraints, make sure that you have adequate help available. Talk to the patient, explaining what's happening and why, and try to calm him down. Have other staff members physically restrain his limbs — one staff member for each limb, if possible. Once the patient has been physically restrained, administer any ordered sedative, then apply the mechanical restraints.

Several types of restraints exist. Know which types your institution has and where they're kept. Soft restraints limit movement to prevent the confused, combative patient from harming himself or others.

The Posey belt and Posey vest have straps that you can tie or lock to a chair or bed. Be sure to apply the Posey vest properly to ensure that it won't slip up and impair the patient's respiration. If you secure the Posey restraints to a chair, choose a heavy chair that won't easily overturn and injure the patient.

You can use cloth wrist restraints to secure a patient's arms to a chair or a bed. Be sure not to apply them too tightly to avoid causing friction burns, skin tears, abrasions, bruises, and impaired circulation.

You may use leather or plastic cuffs for the ankles and wrists to restrain a young, strong, aggressive patient. Depending on the patient's behavior, you may apply these restraints to all limbs (four-point restraints) or to one arm and one leg (two-point restraints), securing them to the bed frame and locking them in place. As with cloth restraints, be careful not to apply these restraints too tightly.

For a patient who fights leather restraints (for example, by bucking violently in the bed), you may use a body net to prevent injury. Secured to the bed frame with numerous straps, the body net confines the patient to the bed and prevents movement. You can also apply a body net

to an ambulatory patient; this allows him to move about but prevents him from hitting or kicking.

Whichever type of restraint you use, be sure to provide proper care for the patient while he's restrained. (See *Caring for a patient in mechanical restraints* for details.)

Be aware that in some cases, physical restraint is a prelude to seclusion — removing a patient to a single room, usually locked and with few furnishings, to reduce the risk of injury to him and others.

*Drug treatment.* As ordered, administer appropriate drugs to control aggressive behavior. These include benzodiazepines, lithium, propranolol, and anticonvulsants.

Short-acting benzodiazepines are used in patients with anxiety-associated agitation. Lithium may be useful in long-term treatment of the emotionally labile, impulsive patient. During lithium therapy, routinely monitor serum lithium levels to ensure therapeutic levels (0.8 to 1.2 mEq/liter).

Propranolol is used for patients with an organic brain injury. Anticonvulsants may be beneficial for some patients with episodic dyscontrol syndrome, rage reactions, hostility, or aggressiveness.

### Evaluation
When evaluating the effectiveness of your interventions, ask yourself these questions:
• Did any injury occur to the patient or to others?
• Was the patient's behavior controlled even though his mood was intense?
• Did I identify aggression at the earliest possible stage and intervene promptly?
• Was the patient's self-esteem maintained?

## Caring for a patient in mechanical restraints

Once a patient's restraints have been secured, you'll need to follow certain steps.

### During the restraint period
• Monitor the patient closely. Offer him food and fluids at frequent intervals, and provide ample opportunities for elimination. Help prevent pressure ulcers by repositioning him regularly, padding bony prominences, and massaging any vulnerable areas.
• Assure the patient that he will be monitored closely. Explain that he'll be released from the restraints when he no longer poses a threat to himself, others, or the environment.
• If appropriate, remove one restraint at a time to allow range-of-motion exercise in an arm or a leg.
• Ensure that all appropriate nursing personnel have keys to remove the restraints in the event of a medical emergency, such as a seizure.

• Monitor circulation to limbs frequently and take measures to prevent impaired circulation, such as not applying restraints too tightly and providing adequate padding.

### Removing restraints
• Make sure that you know and follow hospital policy and state law regarding the duration of restraint.
• Don't remove restraints without sufficient staff present to physically restrain the patient should he become agitated.
• Gradually release a patient in four-point restraints to two-point restraints, removing the restraints on opposite limbs — such as the right leg and left arm. Remove the last two restraints at the same time.
• After restraining a patient, call a staff meeting to discuss what went well and what needs improvement.

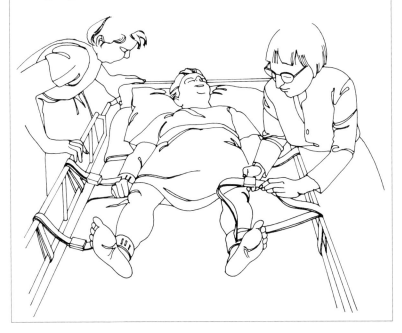

• Did the patient's aggressive behavior decrease?
• Did I follow hospital policy, legal guidelines, and therapeutic principles for verbal intervention, physical restraint, and pharmacologic intervention, if needed?
• Was I able to identify and deal with my own feelings?

Realize that the aggressive patient will test limits. Ideally, he'll begin to express his feelings more directly and use more appropriate coping techniques to deal with stressful situations. When this occurs, provide positive feedback. Don't be discouraged if he regresses to his previous behavior, as long as he can discuss the behavior appropriately.

Keep in mind that any behavioral changes take time. Because the patient may not be hospitalized for the length of time needed to realize these changes, you must provide him with psychiatric, legal, or community health referrals in your discharge planning.

***Requesting a consultation.*** Consult a psychiatrist or psychiatric clinical nurse specialist whenever your "talk-down" techniques prove ineffective. The clinical nurse specialist may be able to communicate with the patient more effectively and help him regain his self-control. If not, the psychiatrist may order drug therapy or mechanical restraints.

# Patient who acts out sexually

Inappropriate sexual behavior may occur when a patient feels a loss of control or a threat to his sexuality.

Such behavior may also be a response to hospitalization and illness, or it may be a chronic problem. Forms of acting out sexually include making obscene or provocative remarks or gestures, exhibiting genitalia, and touching oneself or another person in a sexual manner. Regardless of the form, acting out sexually is always inappropriate and detrimental to a therapeutic relationship between nurse and patient.

### Assessment
To plan effective interventions, you need to explore the patient's behavior and its origins and then assess your own feelings toward him.

***Identifying behavioral patterns and dynamics.*** Assess the nature of the patient's behavior before, during, and after the sexual acting out occurs. Investigate his health history for possible clues to the origins of his behavior.

To help determine the cause of his behavior and identify appropriate problem-solving techniques, explore the following questions:
• Was the behavior present before hospitalization?
• Does the patient exhibit signs of heightened stress, anxiety, or tension before and after the undesirable behavior?
• Does the behavior diminish his anxiety?
• Is the behavior most prominent during a family visit?
• Does his acting out sexually proceed or follow treatments he finds undesirable?

Consider the many possible factors related to the underlying dynamics of acting out sexually. Commonly, inappropriate sexual behavior occurs in a patient who's unsure of his physical attractiveness (for example, a patient who has undergone a colostomy) or his ability to perform sexually (for instance, a patient with diabetes). In other patients, inappropriate sexual behavior may be a coping mechanism aimed at allaying anxiety related to hospitalization.

Be aware that inappropriate sexual behavior sometimes reflects low self-esteem or feelings of inadequacy and inferiority. A patient who cannot cope with socialization or develop relationships may act out sexually in a misguided attempt to establish some sort of relationship.

Early victimization or past sexual abuse may contribute to inappropriate sexual behavior. For instance, an adult who was sexually abused as a child may view behavior deemed by society to be sexually deviant as perfectly normal. Mental illness, personality disorders, dysfunctional family or parent relationships, limit testing, and a need to attract attention can also cause inappropriate sexual behavior.

***Examining your feelings.*** To deal effectively with the patient, you need to examine your own feelings about his behavior. You should identify and confront your feelings, which may include disgust, contempt, indignation, anger, rage, embarrassment, or fear, before attempting to openly discuss with the patient his inappropriate behavior and provide therapeutic interventions.

You should also evaluate your own knowledge of sexual topics. You need to be able to supply correct information, clear up any misconceptions, and avoid giving stereotypical, unhelpful responses to the patient.

## Intervention
Focus your interventions on setting limits on inappropriate sexual be-

havior, conveying understanding and empathy, and making appropriate referrals for more in-depth psychological evaluation and care.

***Setting limits.*** Confront the patient and let him know that his behavior is unacceptable. Tell him that when he acts out sexually, he makes you feel uncomfortable, and then clearly describe the behavior you expect. For example, say to him, "Mr. Johnson, I feel uncomfortable when you make suggestive comments. Please stop it." Ignoring the problem or laughing it off neither benefits the patient nor promotes the development of a therapeutic relationship.

After determining the best plan of action, record it on the nursing care plan. This ensures consistent limit setting by all staff members.

***Conveying understanding and empathy.*** Reassure the patient that you aren't rejecting him personally, just his behavior. Explain that you realize his behavior is an expression of his feelings, and allow him to explore why he feels and acts the way he does. Explore alternative methods of channeling behavior. For instance, when a desire to act out sexually occurs, suggest that he redirect his thoughts or discuss with a staff member his feelings and how they relate to his past experiences. Give positive reinforcement for appropriate behavior.

If necessary, alter your own behavior as well. For example, knock on the patient's door or ask if he's dressed or covered before you enter the room. Also clear up any misunderstandings about the nurse-patient relationship. For instance, help a patient clarify his feelings when he confuses gratitude and admiration for you with feelings of sexual attraction. (See *Dealing with inap-*

## Dealing with inappropriate sexual behavior

To help provide therapeutic intervention for a patient who's acting out sexually, ask yourself these questions:
☐ Am I aware of my own responses? Do I feel uncomfortable, angry, or amused?
☐ During the incident, did I remain calm, objective, and cool, or did I get flustered?
☐ Have I sought emotional support by talking about the incident with my peers or with a psychiatric clinical nurse specialist? Have I asked for advice on how they might have handled the incident differently?
☐ Do I recognize that this behavior may occur again? Have I thought about how I'll deal with the problem if it happens again? Will I resist the temptation to ignore this behavior?
☐ Have I set limits with the patient? Did I tell him which specific behaviors are unacceptable?
☐ Have I explored new ways to cope with the situation?
☐ Have I slowly begun to develop a trusting, open, honest, relationship with the patient? Am I making sure that I don't rush the relationship because this may cause negative behavior?
☐ Am I certain that I'm not blaming myself for the patient's behavior?

propriate sexual behavior for more information on specific interventions.)

***Making appropriate referrals.*** If needed, refer the patient for more in-depth assistance. Consult with a psychiatric clinical nurse specialist, psychiatrist, psychologist, or social worker with specialized training in sex therapy. The patient may need intensive sex education and counsel-

ing, sex therapy, and individual or marital therapy.

### Evaluation
Weigh the effectiveness of your interventions by exploring the patient's behavioral changes. Ask yourself these questions:
• Can the patient express an understanding of why his behavior was unacceptable?
• Can he control his behavior?
• Does he take responsibility for his actions?
• Can he correctly describe the feelings of the victims of his behavior?
• Is he using adaptive coping mechanisms?
• Did he feel that the care he received helped him meet his health care goals?
• Was my nursing assessment of the patient's sexuality complete, accurate, and done in a professional manner?
• Did I explore and handle my own feelings and values about sexuality appropriately?

***Requesting a consultation.*** You may want to consult with a psychiatrist or psychiatric clinical nurse specialist to help you deal with your own feelings and to help plan an effective strategy for dealing with a patient who acts out sexually.

# Malingering patient

Malingering involves intentional feigning or exaggeration of physical or psychological symptoms for ulterior motives. A malingerer deceives others — but not himself — about his symptoms and in so doing may receive some secondary gain. For example, he may receive financial

## Distinguishing malingering from psychological disorders

In some patients, you may need to distinguish malingering from certain psychological disorders, such as:
• factitious disorder with physical symptoms (Münchausen syndrome). The person seeks recurrent hospitalization for physical symptoms, which may involve any body system. However, unlike the malingerer, he has no external incentives for experiencing symptoms. Commonly, he has a history of incarceration and drug problems.
• factitious disorder with psychological symptoms. The person intentionally feigns psychological symptoms to receive treatment and become a patient.

He has no external incentives for feigning these symptoms.
• conversion disorder. The person experiences alteration or loss of physical functioning, suggesting a physical illness, but with no organic cause. Symptoms are related to an underlying emotional conflict, but the person is unaware of the disorder's psychological origin.
• somatization disorder. The person has a history of multiple physical complaints with no organic cause. Onset is usually before age 30. Symptoms aren't necessarily associated with a panic attack and may require medical attention and treatment.

compensation or drugs, he may have an excuse for not working, or he may somehow evade criminal prosecution. Commonly misdiagnosed as numerous physical illnesses, malingering wastes millions of dollars each year in health care costs.

### Assessment

Suspect malingering in a patient with one or more of the following:
• medicolegal reason for hospitalization, such as referral by a lawyer
• marked discrepancy between reported symptoms and observed behavior
• poor cooperation with diagnostic evaluation or failure to adhere to the treatment regimen
• antisocial personality disorders, commonly marked by a history of school, employment, legal, and marital difficulties
• vague or contradictory health history information
• little or no symptomatic relief from known effective treatment, or some improvement initially but reappear-

ance of symptoms as the time for discharge grows near.

Obtaining an accurate health history from a malingerer may be impossible because secrecy is in his best interest. The malingerer typically uses out-of-town doctors, different pharmacies, and various hospitals to cover his trail.

Further complicating assessment is the fact that a malingerer commonly exhibits real symptoms. For example, a patient complaining of GI bleeding may indeed have blood in his stool and a low hemoglobin level because he inflicted injury to himself to produce these symptoms.

A malingerer also may use alcohol and other drugs to produce symptoms. For example, he may use stimulants such as amphetamines or caffeine to cause insomnia or restlessness; hallucinogens such as LSD or mescaline to produce altered levels of consciousness and perception; analgesics such as morphine to produce euphoria; and hypnotics or alcohol to cause lethargy.

In some patients, you may need to differentiate malingering from actual disorders that mimic it. (See *Distinguishing malingering from psychological disorders,* page 51.)

***Examining your feelings.*** A malingering patient may elicit from you feelings of frustration, anger, or contempt. Before you can develop a therapeutic relationship with the patient, you need to identify and deal with your own negative feelings.

### Intervention
You may find it difficult to intervene effectively for a malingering patient because he will typically refuse psychiatric consultation. Avoid power struggles, heated verbal exchanges, and punitive interventions. Confrontation may cause the patient to act out, sometimes aggressively, in an attempt to prove that he's ill.

Consult with the patient's doctor, a psychiatric clinical nurse specialist, or a psychiatrist to develop a consistent, effective care plan. Explain to the patient that his complaints don't call for the treatment he's requesting or demanding. Be aware that he may become angry when confronted and may leave to find another institution or caregiver who will provide the treatment he has requested. Eventually, however, a malingerer will exhaust all his options, at which time attempts to confront him should be more effective.

You'll find it almost impossible to explore the underlying causes for malingering because it's conscious behavior, and the patient has taken pains to conceal the reasons for it. The reasons he gives may be so far from the truth that discovering the real reason is virtually impossible.

Encourage the malingerer to assume responsibility for his own physical care to minimize the secondary gain of dependency on his caregiver. Responsibility fosters continued independence and improves self-esteem. Assertiveness training and stress reduction techniques may help the patient face stressors in a positive way. However, learning these techniques may require more time than is available during his hospitalization. If you feel these techniques would be helpful, refer the patient to community facilities that offer these services.

### Evaluation
Because you can never be completely certain whether or not a patient is malingering, you'll find evaluating his progress toward adaptive behavior difficult. Typically, a malingerer continues his behavior until he has exhausted all avenues that might fulfill his needs, accepts responsibility for his behavior, and chooses to change it.

***Requesting a consultation.*** You may find it beneficial to consult with a psychiatrist or a psychiatric clinical nurse specialist during assessment. Psychological testing may confirm a diagnosis of malingering and an underlying personality disorder. Unfortunately, most malingerers won't submit to testing.

You'll also want to consult with the psychiatrist or psychiatric clinical nurse specialist before confronting the patient, to help determine his potential for self-abuse.

# Obsessive-compulsive patient

Obsessions are involuntary recurrent and persistent ideas, thoughts,

# Assessing the obsessive-compulsive patient

If you suspect obsessive-compulsive behavior in a patient, ask yourself the following questions:
• Does the patient demonstrate compulsive, ritualistic behavior, such as frequent hand washing, checking, counting, touching, or doing and undoing?
• Does he state that this behavior causes either physical or emotional discomfort?
• Does he dread not being able to perform the behavior to eliminate negative thoughts?
• Does he feel his symptoms become more difficult to live with during times of stress?
• Does he overemphasize neatness and cleanliness?
• Does he have unrealistically high standards for himself?
• Is he estranged from his family or experiencing difficulty at work because of his behavior?
• What does the patient fear?

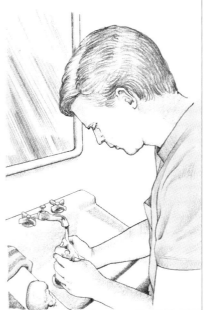

images, or impulses that invade a person's consciousness despite attempts to ignore or suppress them. Compulsions, on the other hand, are repetitive and seemingly purposeful behaviors performed according to certain rules or in a stereotyped fashion, aimed at producing or preventing some future event or situation.

In many cases, the obsessive-compulsive patient knows that his obsessional thoughts are irrational, but he continues the ritualistic, compulsive behavior to decrease anxiety. Despite evidence to the contrary, he denies that his behavior causes distress and interferes with social functioning.

Obsessive-compulsive behavior may be more common in the general population than in a psychiatric setting. Obsessions and compulsions develop normally in childhood. And most normal adults exhibit some degree of compulsive behavior when faced with a threat or risk. But no clear-cut theories explain why some people go on to develop obsessive-compulsive disorder and others do not.

In most cases, people with obsessive-compulsive disorder seek treatment only when their behavior causes physical symptoms or psychological stress. In the hospital, these patients can be especially challenging because their ritualistic behavior can interfere with hospital routine.

## Assessment
If you suspect that your patient has obsessive-compulsive disorder, focus your assessment on identifying characteristic symptom clusters. (See *Assessing the obsessive-compulsive patient,* page 53.) You may detect four major symptom clusters occurring alone or in various combinations. Many of these patients describe obsessions about dirt and contamination and compulsive behavior involving ritualistic hand washing (in some cases, to the point of causing skin problems), which usually lowers anxiety. The patient may be more fearful of self-contamination than of contaminating others. When confronted, he usually can recognize that his compulsive behavior is irrational, but he can't stop doing it.

A second cluster of symptoms involves compulsive checking, with obsessional thoughts revolving around a fear of violence. An affected person worries that catastrophe may result from his failure to maintain constant vigilance. Such a compulsive checker lives as if he's a guilty party in search of a crime. However, he usually can hide his symptoms and present a socially acceptable picture.

A third cluster of symptoms, pure obsessions, involves repetitive intrusive thoughts, usually sexual or aggressive and always associated with impulses or fearful images. Although to you these thoughts may seem relatively neutral, to the patient they're a major source of anxiety. Despite aggressive impulses, however, the patient may be able to resist the compulsion to hurt himself or others by imagining every possible consequence of acting on the obsession.

The rarest and most disabling symptom cluster involves an obses-

sive slowness. An example of this would be a patient who takes an hour to brush his teeth or 2 hours to eat a meal. This cluster may be associated with adolescent eating disorders, such as anorexia nervosa or bulimia. In these disorders, social pressures to conform to an "ideal" body weight, combined with the person's predisposition for obsessive-compulsive disorder, produces symptoms. The adolescent becomes obsessed with eating and thinking about food, counting calories, and exercising. In extreme cases, these behaviors may occupy most of the adolescent's time.

In many patients, you may detect obsessive-compulsive behavior combined with other psychiatric illnesses. Most commonly, you'll note features of depression, phobias, or borderline personality disorders.

## Intervention
Interventions for an obsessive-compulsive patient include establishing goals, building a therapeutic relationship, administering medications, assisting with behavioral therapy, and making referrals.

*Establishing goals.* Short-term goals for an obsessive-compulsive patient include identifying stressors, reducing anxiety, encouraging open discussion of feelings, promoting independence, decreasing possible aggression, and improving self-esteem. The long-term goal is eliminating the need for compulsive behavior by decreasing anxiety caused by obsessive thoughts.

*Building a therapeutic relationship.* When caring for a patient with obsessive-compulsive disorder, follow these guidelines:
• Don't keep the patient from performing the compulsive behavior —

unless it's self-destructive — and allow time for rituals. Prohibiting these behaviors will exacerbate his anxiety, possibly to the level of panic.

• Anticipate and meet the patient's needs. For instance, you should perform procedures at scheduled times. This can help increase the patient's sense of security by reducing his anxiety and reinforcing his worth.

• Don't call undue attention to the patient's rituals. He already believes they're foolish.

• Shield the patient from ridicule, which lowers self-esteem and increases anxiety.

• Protect the patient from injury caused by ritualistic behavior. For example, provide frequent skin care for a patient who performs excessive hand washing.

• As the patient becomes more comfortable and involved in unit routines, gradually reduce the time allowed for rituals and encourage adaptive substitute activities.

• Help the patient identify anxiety-provoking situations or events that trigger rituals.

• As ordered, teach the patient ways to interrupt his ritualistic behaviors. For example, teach him to snap a rubber band on his wrist to remind himself to try to stop his obsessive thoughts.

• Provide positive feedback for adaptive behavior, which encourages the behavior and can increase self-esteem. Also, point out that making mistakes is acceptable and that he needn't strive for perfection.

• Avoid nurse-patient power struggles, which lead to anxiety in the patient and frustration in the staff.

***Administering drug therapy.*** As ordered, administer medications to treat obsessive-compulsive behavior. Expect to give such drugs as tri-

cyclic antidepressants and lithium, which have shown limited success, and newer drugs, such as the potent serotonin uptake inhibitors clomipramine (Anafranil) and fluoxetine (Prozac), which seem more promising. Many patients receiving drug therapy report fewer obsessive thoughts, an increased ability to resist ritualistic behavior, and a return to a more normal level of social functioning.

Be aware, however, that drug therapy is not without certain drawbacks. A long course of treatment — typically longer than 6 weeks — is required, making the patient prone to adverse drug reactions. Severe adverse reactions may necessitate discontinuing drug therapy, and a high relapse rate occurs within weeks after the drug is discontinued. What's more, for some patients, taking the medication actually becomes the focus for obsessional preoccupation. This may be severe enough to preclude drug treatment.

***Aiding with behavioral therapy.*** You may care for a patient receiving behavioral therapy combined with drug therapy and psychotherapy. Depending on the severity of the disorder, behavioral therapy takes between 1 and 6 months and has two aspects. In exposure therapy, the patient is encouraged to come into prolonged contact with discomforting cues that bring on the rituals. Then he's prevented from engaging in the ritualistic behavior until his anxiety and the urge to perform the rituals subside.

In another approach, the patient is also exposed to discomforting cues but substitutes passive avoidance behavior patterns for ritualistic behavior. This behavior controls the anxiety associated with situations that cause fear and leaves the patient believing that avoiding the precipitating situations protects him from harm.

***Making appropriate referrals.*** Because the patient's length of stay in the hospital may not be long enough to accomplish all of these goals — particularly the long-term goals — you and the patient can only begin to work toward accomplishing them. Depending on the patient's degree of physical and psychological distress and his motivation, you can make psychiatric referrals while he's an inpatient or after discharge.

### Evaluation
Because complete remission of obsessive-compulsive behavior usually isn't the goal of treatment, evaluation focuses on determining whether obsessive-compulsive symptoms and the patient's anxiety have diminished. Through a combination of drug and behavioral therapy, as well as psychotherapy, a patient may be able to confront what triggers his anxiety and then delay, diminish, or even completely stop his ritualistic behavior. Behavioral therapy usually isn't effective for a severely depressed or delusional patient, or for a patient who fails to comply with therapy.

Of course, you won't be able to see the outcomes of long-term therapy in a general hospital setting. You'll only be able to see that the patient has suffered no physical harm from performing ritualistic acts during his stay in the hospital.

***Requesting a consultation.*** You may find that referral for psychiatric evaluation is most beneficial to patients whose ritualistic behavior has impaired their social functioning. At the same time, working with a psychiatrist or psychiatric clinical nurse specialist can be very helpful in developing effective care plans.

# Dependent patient

A universal personality trait and an essential aspect of every human being's development, dependency is normal and even expected in a patient. To receive treatment, a patient allows caregivers to make many decisions for him, and dependency can help him cope with his illness or injury. Normally though, with support and encouragement he will, after an appropriate period, resume his independence and undertake self-care activities.

But dependency can become a problem for some patients. Many people have underlying tendencies toward dependency, learned in childhood, that they usually can keep under control. But sometimes these tendencies surface during periods of separation from a parent, sibling, or spouse. And some patients refuse to relinquish the role of a sick person after an appropriate period of time and strongly resist taking responsibility for their own care. This behavior may stem from various factors, including undesirable outcomes of past decisions, feelings of helplessness, perceived convenience, or maladaptive coping mechanisms. (See *Understanding dependent behavior* for more information.)

A dependent patient lacks self-confidence and cannot function well independently. He may mask this problem with an overly confident, optimistic, and outgoing demeanor or by being overly solicitous and compliant. In an attempt to avoid the risk of becoming self-sufficient, the patient allows others to become responsible for his life. For example, he may let caregivers make every major decision for him.

## Assessment

During your assessment, keep in mind that a dependent patient may exhibit a wide range of behaviors and express various emotions, including:

• feelings of being overwhelmed
• tenseness
• depression
• guilt and feelings of inadequacy
• talkativeness
• insistent or clinging behavior
• passivity
• helplessness
• aggressive, antisocial behavior
• paranoid interactions with others.

During your assessment, explore the following questions:

• How does the patient function outside the hospital? In what type of role?
• Does he have adequate support systems? What are they?
• How does he feel about being hospitalized?
• Does he have a history of multiple hospitalizations?
• How does he care for himself on a daily basis?
• Does he feel inadequate, depressed, or hopeless?
• What physical, psychological, and environmental changes may contribute to his dependency?

Remember that the dependent patient wants you to be near him. To accomplish this, he may become overly solicitous and talkative in an attempt to trigger guilt in you if you leave him. Another patient may tearfully request that you stay nearby. Note any such behavior.

Also be alert for self-destructive threats or behavior, which may oc-

## Understanding dependent behavior

Dependency is characterized by three related features:

• strong emotional reliance on others — for example, a child or adolescent prone to separation anxiety or an elderly patient who doesn't want to feel alone and helpless and who constantly makes demands (such as for more water, another pillow, or backrubs)
• poor self-confidence, often accompanied by submissive behavior — for example, a patient who won't alert the nurse to his discomfort or pain for fear of eliciting anger, criticism, or abandonment
• indecisiveness, avoidance of autonomy, and difficulty initiating or completing activities — for example, a patient who refuses to learn self-care procedures that he's physically able to perform.

cur as a patient becomes increasingly desperate for attention.

Finally, remember that any move toward independence is also apt to reactivate the patient's dependency needs. This is especially true in the long-term patient who's ready for discharge. Note any complaints of sudden aches and pains or such statements as "I'm not ready to go home" or "Are you sure I can tell when my blood sugar is getting too high?"

***Examining your feelings.*** Evaluate how you react to the dependent patient. If you find yourself rejecting or avoiding him, you may be fostering his dependency. Try to resolve any feelings of anger or frustration that can interfere with developing a therapeutic relationship with the patient.

## Intervention

Focus your nursing interventions for a dependent patient on establishing realistic goals and promoting the patient's independence.

*Setting goals.* Set attainable short-term goals for patient care. Examples include helping the patient to express his feelings, gain insight into his behavior, become involved in self-care, and make some independent decisions. Also consider such long-term goals as helping the patient develop means to promote wellness, eliminate physical symptoms that precipitate his hospitalization, and develop new, adaptive coping mechanisms, such as assertiveness.

*Encouraging independence.* At first, give the patient all the care and attention he requests. Don't force him to assume self-care responsibilities before he's ready. Strive to develop a trusting relationship. When you feel that the patient trusts you, talk to him about his behavior, and gradually encourage him to make some decisions for himself and begin performing some self-care measures. Consult with the patient when planning his daily schedule to develop mutually agreeable priorities.

Keep in mind that pressuring the patient to make decisions or perform self-care too quickly can trigger anxiety. On the other hand, avoiding the patient or ignoring his requests can only lead to increased dependency.

Provide positive comments on the patient's decision-making ability and judgment. Demonstrate empathy when confronting the patient about inappropriate requests.

Teach the patient to communicate directly and honestly and to become more assertive. Point out to the patient that at certain times and in certain situations, confusion, anger, and uncertainty are appropriate responses.

Finally, don't withdraw your support too quickly as the patient begins exhibiting signs of increased independence. Doing so may cause the patient to worry about abandonment and lose confidence in your relationship.

Make certain that all staff members are aware of planned interventions, and keep the patient care plan up-to-date. During discharge planning, explain the patient's dependency problems and his progress to future caregivers. Assist family members in understanding the patient's problem, and discuss their role in encouraging his independence.

## Evaluation

Depending on the patient's length of stay in the hospital, he should begin to assume some self-care activities and independent decision making. Determine whether the short-term goals have been met or whether the patient at least has made any progress toward achieving them.

Evaluate your own responses to the patient, asking yourself these questions:
• Have I established a caring, trusting relationship with the patient?
• Have I placed the relationship in jeopardy as a result of any of my actions?
• How do I feel about caring for this patient?
• Am I providing enough positive reinforcement and attention?
• Do I blame myself for the patient's failure to achieve goals?

For a patient in a general hospital setting, you can hope to achieve short-term goals. But long-term goals, which require more time and support, may be achieved only after the patient's discharge.

**Requesting a consultation** You may find that consulting with a psychiatric clinical nurse specialist may help you sort out your own feelings and plan appropriate interventions for the patient. Scheduled staff conferences to go over the patient's progress and to discuss suggestions for change can be invaluable. If the patient has continuing dependency needs that interfere with his ability to function, psychiatric consultation may be needed and therapy may be started while he's in the hospital.

## Suggested readings

Breier, A., et al. "Controllable and Uncontrollable Stress in Humans: Alterations in Mood and Neuroendocrine and Psychophysiological Function," *American Journal of Psychiatry* 144(11):1419-25, November 1987.

Cosgray, R.E., and Fawley, R.W. "Could it Be Ganser's Syndrome?" *Archives of Psychiatric Nursing* 3(4):241-45, August 1989.

Davidhizar, R.E. "Handling Manipulation," *Health Care Supervisor* 8(3):37-44, April 1990.

*Diagnostic and Statistical Manual of Mental Disorders,* 3rd ed., revised. Washington, D.C.: American Psychiatric Association, 1987.

Fletcher, K.R. "Restraints Should Be a Last Resort," *RN* 53(1):52-56, January, 1990.

Greist, J.H. "Treating the Anxiety: Therapeutic Options in Obsessive-Compulsive Disorder," *Journal of Clinical Psychiatry* 51(11, Suppl):29-34, November 1990.

Gruber, M., et al. "Trying to Care for a Great Pretender," *Nursing87* 17(5):76-80, May 1987.

Ingersoll, S.L., and Patton, S.O. *Treating Perpetrators of Sexual Abuse.* Lexington, Mass.: Lexington Books, 1990.

Insel, T.R. "New Pharmacologic Approaches to Obsessive-Compulsive Disorder," *Journal of Clinical Psychiatry* 51(10, Suppl):47-51, October 1990.

Rothenberg, A. "Adolescence and Eating Disorder: The Obsessive-Compulsive Syndrome," *Psychiatric Clinics of North America* 13(3):469-88, September 1990.

Stuart, G.W, and Sundeen, S.J. *Principles and Practice of Psychiatric Nursing,* 4th ed. St. Louis: Mosby-Year Book, Inc., 1991.

Turnbull, J.M. "Anxiety and Physical Illness in the Elderly," *Journal of Clinical Psychiatry* 50(11, Suppl):40-45, November 1989.

Varcarolis, E.M. *Foundations of Psychiatric Mental Health Nursing.* Philadelphia: W.B. Saunders Co., 1990.

Venn, E.S., and Derdeyn, A.D. "Working with a Difficult Adolescent," *Journal of Psychosocial Nursing and Mental Health Services* 26(6):28-33, June 1988.

Vogel, C.H., et al. "Exploring the Concept of Manipulation in Psychiatric Settings," *Archives of Psychiatric Nursing* 1(6):429-35, December 1987.

Wise, M.G., and Taylor, S.E. "Anxiety and Mood Disorders in Medically Ill Patients," *Journal of Clinical Psychiatry* 51(Suppl):27-32, January 1990.

Zanarini, M.C., et al. "Discriminating Borderline Personality Disorder from other Axis II Disorders," *American Journal of Psychiatry* 147(2):161-67, February 1990.

# 4

# ANXIETY

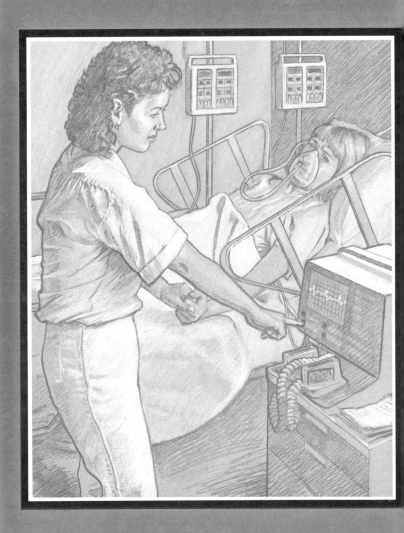

People of all ages experience some form of anxiety in their everyday lives. Such anxiety may result from any number of immediate causes—a threat of deprivation or loss of control, a decreased ability to function, a fear of disapproval and rejection, low self-esteem, or frustration, for example. But hospital patients run a special risk of developing anxiety because of the physical and emotional stress associated with hospitalization and illness.

In this chapter, you'll learn to assess an anxious patient and help him identify what's triggering his anxiety—an important first step toward conquering it. You'll also read about how to perform immediate interventions and begin long-term management. Plus, you'll review how to evaluate your patient's progress following your interventions. But first, sharpen your understanding of anxiety by reading about the different types as well as the psychophysiologic effects and possible underlying causes.

# Understanding anxiety

A universal experience, anxiety can be defined as a vague, uneasy feeling, or as apprehension or tension stemming from the anticipation of danger from an unknown or unspecified source. Physiologically, the body reacts the same way to anxiety as it does to fear. However, anxiety results from a real or perceived threat, whereas fear is a reaction to a specific danger.

Anxiety can occur whenever a person believes that his life or self-esteem is threatened. A threat to his life may include a real or perceived interference with basic needs, such as food, warmth, or drink. A threat to his self-esteem may be more obscure because each person's sense of self is unique. Such a threat may take several forms, including unmet expectations that are important to personal integrity, unmet needs for prestige and status, guilt associated with differences between how the person may view himself and his actual behavior, the loss of an important role such as that of spouse or employee, or an inability to gain approval, respect, or recognition from one's peers.

Anxiety warns a person that something is wrong. Mild anxiety may increase a person's alertness and motivate him to examine what's wrong, make changes, and move ahead. But anxiety can also immobilize a person. As anxiety intensifies or lingers, it becomes harmful—even pathologic.

Pathologic anxiety is an emotional illness characterized by intense fear and symptoms associated with the autonomic nervous system, such as palpitations, tachycardia, dizziness, and tremor. The anxiety is considered pathologic because it occurs in response to stressors that the average person can usually cope with and because the patient concentrates all his actions on trying to control the anxiety.

## Types of anxiety
Anxiety disorders are classified into five basic types: panic disorders, generalized anxiety disorders, phobias, obsessive-compulsive disorder, and posttraumatic stress disorder. Almost every hospitalized patient experiences some anxiety, and many have one of these anxiety disorders. So you should be prepared to manage all five types.

CHECKLIST

## Reviewing common phobias

Resulting from an intense fear of a specific object, situation, or activity, a phobia can trigger a reaction ranging from mild anxiety to panic. The list below gives the clinical names and brief definitions of some common phobias you may encounter.
- □ *Acrophobia*—fear of heights
- □ *Agoraphobia*—fear of open spaces
- □ *Astraphobia*—fear of electrical storms
- □ *Claustrophobia*—fear of closed spaces
- □ *Glossophobia*—fear of talking
- □ *Hematophobia*—fear of blood
- □ *Hydrophobia*—fear of water
- □ *Monophobia*—fear of being alone
- □ *Mysophobia*—fear of germs and dirt
- □ *Pyrophobia*—fear of fire
- □ *Zoophobia*—fear of animals

**Panic disorders.** In a panic disorder, the feeling of terror is so severe that the patient can no longer function normally. A panic attack may occur suddenly, intensify, and then subside in a few minutes. The patient may feel that he's having a heart attack, reporting such symptoms as heart pounding, dyspnea, dizziness, and light-headedness.

**Generalized anxiety disorders.** A patient with a generalized anxiety disorder lives in a constant state of worry, often over matters others would consider trivial. He dreads making a mistake and has poor concentration and difficulty with decision making. Typically, he worries about the physical symptoms that he's experiencing.

**Phobias.** An irrational, intense fear of an object, situation, or activity, a phobia can be grouped into one of three classes: agoraphobia, simple phobias, and social phobias.

*Agoraphobia* is a fear of being in an open, crowded, or public place, where escape may be difficult or help not available in case of sudden incapacitation. Panic attacks are commonly associated with this phobia.

*Simple phobias,* which are common, are associated with a fear or avoidance of a single object, activity, or situation. A simple phobia usually doesn't interfere significantly in a person's life.

*Social phobias* involve the fear of not being able to function in public—for instance, a fear of doing or saying something that's socially unacceptable. A social phobia can lead to substance abuse to help relieve anxiety. (See *Reviewing common phobias.*)

**Obsessive-compulsive disorder.** An obsession is a recurring thought that the patient can't voluntarily remove from his consciousness. A compulsion is a recurring, irresistible impulse to perform some action that temporarily relieves the impulse, thus reducing anxiety. The patient doesn't want to repeat the thought or action but feels compelled to do so. These behaviors may be combined or may occur separately.

**Posttraumatic stress disorder.** This form of anxiety can occur after any psychologically traumatic event—an assault, a war, a rape, or an earthquake, for example. In acute posttraumatic stress disorder, symptoms occur within 6 months of the trauma. In the chronic form, symptoms either are delayed for more than 6 months or have lasted for 6 months.

## Psychophysiologic effects

Anxiety can affect a patient physically, emotionally, intellectually, spiritually, and socially. A patient may handle mild anxiety unconsciously with few observable signs. As anxiety becomes moderate, he'll seek ways to avoid or cope with it.

Coping mechanisms help the patient neutralize, counteract, or deny the anxiety. Typical coping mechanisms include crying, eating, sleeping, yawning, laughing, cursing, performing physical exercise, daydreaming, and engaging in oral behavior, such as smoking or drinking. The patient also may limit close relationships to those in which he feels most comfortable.

Moderate to severe anxiety causes a greater threat to the ego and requires more energy to counteract. Typically, the patient's reaction will be task-oriented or ego-oriented.

In a *task-oriented reaction*, a person tries to deal with the threatening situation. Common task-oriented reactions include attack, withdrawal, and compromise. Each type can be either constructive or destructive.

An attack reaction focuses on meeting anxiety head-on. Constructive attack reactions involve a problem-solving approach, whereas destructive attack reactions may involve anger and hostility and represent negative-aggressive behavior.

Psychological or physical withdrawal focuses on separating oneself from the source of anxiety. A person withdraws psychologically from a threatening situation by admitting defeat, lowering his expectations, or becoming apathetic. He withdraws physically by removing himself from the situation that produces the threat.

When a person compromises, he changes his way of doing things, substitutes goals, or sacrifices certain aspects of his personal needs. Although usually constructive, compromise can be destructive if it harms the person's self-concept.

In place of a task-oriented reaction, a person may instead use an *ego-oriented reaction* (also called an ego-defense mechanism). This type of reaction can take the form of such defense mechanisms as denial, repression, projection, and reaction formation. Such a reaction protects the person from anxiety and low self-esteem, but it also can interfere with rational decision making.

***Physical effects.*** The autonomic nervous system produces physiologic changes associated with anxiety. The sympathetic nervous system responds to a threat by releasing epinephrine, causing increases in heart and respiratory rates, arterial pressure, glycogenolysis (glucose production by the liver), and blood glucose levels. The parasympathetic nervous system responds by attempting to conserve energy. (See *How the body responds to anxiety,* page 64.)

***Emotional changes.*** A patient reveals his emotional response to anxiety through his words and actions. He may tell you he feels uneasy, on edge, tense, worried, or restless. Or he may say he feels as if something bad is about to happen. Also, a patient may describe feelings of jealousy, self-deprecation, worthlessness, or contempt. And he may appear angry, bored, irritable, impatient, fearful, sad, helpless, or depressed. These emotional responses unconsciously help reduce his anxiety.

***Intellectual changes.*** Moderate to severe anxiety affects cognitive function, producing changes in per-

# How the body responds to anxiety

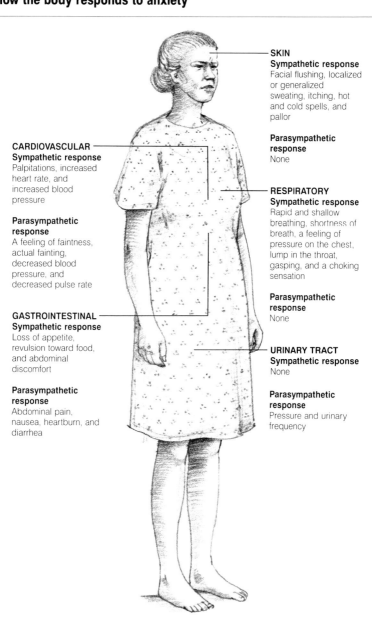

**SKIN**
**Sympathetic response**
Facial flushing, localized or generalized sweating, itching, hot and cold spells, and pallor

**Parasympathetic response**
None

**CARDIOVASCULAR**
**Sympathetic response**
Palpitations, increased heart rate, and increased blood pressure

**Parasympathetic response**
A feeling of faintness, actual fainting, decreased blood pressure, and decreased pulse rate

**RESPIRATORY**
**Sympathetic response**
Rapid and shallow breathing, shortness of breath, a feeling of pressure on the chest, lump in the throat, gasping, and a choking sensation

**Parasympathetic response**
None

**GASTROINTESTINAL**
**Sympathetic response**
Loss of appetite, revulsion toward food, and abdominal discomfort

**Parasympathetic response**
Abdominal pain, nausea, heartburn, and diarrhea

**URINARY TRACT**
**Sympathetic response**
None

**Parasympathetic response**
Pressure and urinary frequency

ception, memory, orientation, judgment and insight, thought content, and communication. As anxiety increases, perception of environmental stimuli decreases until the perceptual field becomes closed or distorted. Memory also diminishes, making the patient unable to recall thoughts or activities, or to retain new ones.

As anxiety grows more severe, the patient's sense of time and place becomes distorted. His judgment becomes impaired, decreasing his insight, decision-making capability, and ability to think abstractly. His attention span decreases, and selective inattention causes him to focus on scattered details. His concentration also decreases, making him unable to understand or follow directions.

As anxiety increases, so does the patient's use of such defense mechanisms as projection, denial, and rationalization. He also may exhibit certain communication patterns, such as pressured speech, blocking, excessive talkativeness, stammering, and rumination.

*Spiritual changes.* As increasing anxiety interferes with the patient's ability to think clearly, make decisions, and feel secure, he may question previously held beliefs and values. Feelings of helplessness and worthlessness can lead to despair. And the patient may find less satisfaction in spiritual or religious activities.

He may also begin to question whether life has any meaning. And he may express a fear of the future and a fear of death.

*Social changes.* Anxiety can disrupt a person's ability to function socially. For instance, an anxious person may try to gain security by talking at great length and in great detail to anyone who will listen. Or he may withdraw from others because of low self-esteem and fear of being rebuffed. Both reactions can increase anxiety.

Excessive, indiscriminate talking may alienate family and friends, decreasing social contact and family and peer support. Excessive use of coping mechanisms, such as denial, projection, rationalization, anger, or withdrawal, can also alienate family and friends.

## Theories on anxiety disorders

You won't find complete agreement on just what causes anxiety disorders. But according to four major theories, anxiety may result from psychodynamic, interpersonal, behavioral, and biological causes.

*Psychodynamic theory.* This theory suggests that anxiety stems from a conflict between the superego and the id. Such a conflict may occur, for instance, when a patient experiences impulses that are unacceptable to him or to others. Anxiety triggers the superego to repress these negative impulses. If repression isn't successful, the patient turns to other defense mechanisms. If these, in turn, don't reduce or contain anxiety, the patient develops symptoms of anxiety disorder.

*Interpersonal theory.* According to this theory, anxiety arises from a fear of disapproval and rejection, possibly stemming from the early bond between mother and child. In children, separation from the mother, concern about parental approval, and developmental traumas all produce anxiety. In adults, anxiety may strike when a person perceives or fears disapproval or loss of love from another person. Typically,

## Physical disorders associated with anxiety

Anxiety results from some physical disorders, and it exacerbates others. Here are some common examples:

**Cardiovascular disorders**
☐ Arrhythmias
☐ Cardiomyopathies
☐ Congestive heart failure
☐ Coronary insufficiency
☐ Mitral valve prolapse
☐ Myocardial infarction

**Endocrine disorders**
☐ Adrenal insufficiency
☐ Carcinoid syndrome
☐ Cushing's syndrome
☐ Hyperparathyroidism
☐ Hyperthyroidism
☐ Hypoglycemia
☐ Hypothyroidism

**Gastrointestinal disorders**
☐ Colitis
☐ Irritable bowel syndrome
☐ Peptic ulcer disease

**Metabolic disorders**
☐ Hypocalcemia
☐ Hypokalemia
☐ Hyponatremia

**Neurologic disorders**
☐ Essential tremor
☐ Huntington's chorea
☐ Lupus cerebritis
☐ Multiple sclerosis
☐ Parkinson's disease
☐ Seizure disorders
☐ Vestibular dysfunction

**Respiratory disorders**
☐ Asthma
☐ Chronic obstructive pulmonary disease
☐ Hyperventilation syndrome
☐ Pneumothorax
☐ Pulmonary edema
☐ Pulmonary embolism

a highly anxious patient will also have low self-esteem, and a discrepancy will exist between his perceived and ideal visions of himself.

***Behavioral theory.*** This theory holds that anxiety is a learned response to past unpleasant experiences—those of the patient, his family, or his friends. For instance, a child may copy a parent's anxious reaction to a particular type of situation.

Behavioral theorists believe that anxiety can either motivate or result from behaviors. Anxiety occurs when a person faces two opposing forces and must decide whether to approach the desired force or avoid the undesired one. For instance, a patient may experience anxiety while deciding whether to have surgery, which may alleviate uncomfortable symptoms (desired) but which will also be painful in the immediate postoperative period (undesired).

***Biological theory.*** A patient's general health affects his predisposition to anxiety. Typically, anxiety accompanies certain physical disorders and is associated with others, including hyperthyroidism, hypoglycemia, and severe pulmonary disease. Anxiety may also exacerbate some disorders, such as hypertension, heart disease, and peptic ulcer. (See *Physical disorders associated with anxiety*.)

Threats to physical integrity and function commonly trigger anxiety. For instance, a patient facing a debilitating physical disorder may wonder how he'll cope with associated pain, restricted activity, financial demands, the resumption of employment and usual routines, and the responses of family members and co-workers. And a terminally ill patient will normally experience anxiety as he faces the loss of his job, the loss of his role in the family, the loss of his physical function, and his eventual death.

Hospitalization also can produce anxiety. Besides the emotional response a hospitalized patient has to his medical problems, he may feel dehumanized by the health care system's rapid pace and advanced technology. Hospitalization can cut off his usual means of maintaining self-esteem. Furthermore, he may be frightened by the loss of control over his body and his environment because of his illness. Forfeiting his daily routine and adapting to the hospital's schedule also may cause him anxiety.

Medications also contribute to anxiety. Drug interactions and adverse reactions can act as toxic stressors, diminishing cognitive function and thus increasing anxiety.

Finally, a patient's overall mental status affects his susceptibility to anxiety. Confusion and memory loss — commonly associated with such disorders as hypoxia and early Alzheimer's disease — frequently bring on anxiety.

---

## Assessment

When a patient shows signs and symptoms of anxiety, you must determine whether he's reacting normally to a perceived threat from a medical disorder or treatment; whether his reaction results from a psychiatric disorder, such as depression; or whether he has a primary anxiety disorder, such as a phobia. After you've identified the nature of the patient's anxiety, determine its severity. Is it mild, moderate, or se-

vere? Is the patient panicking? Remember, anxiety isn't static. Its severity will fluctuate, so you'll need to reassess the patient frequently.

The next step is to help the patient recognize his anxiety and anticipate situations that trigger it. Then you'll help him to identify appropriate ways of coping with his anxiety.

Keep in mind that anxiety is contagious, and don't allow your patient's anxiety to disturb your composure during the assessment. To manage an anxious or fearful patient most effectively, discuss the situation openly with him. Ask him if he's feeling anxious, and encourage him to describe his feelings. Usually, he'll relax somewhat, and you'll be able to proceed more comfortably with the interview.

### Physical assessment

Examine the patient for signs of anxiety not related to his physical illness. In a patient with *mild anxiety*, you may see such signs as increased heart rate, blood pressure, respiratory rate, and muscle tone. This patient also may have decreased salivation, dilated pupils, and cold skin and limbs. He may report insomnia and demonstrate mild tension-relieving behaviors, such as nail biting, finger or foot tapping, and fidgeting. If anxiety causes hyperventilation, he may report shortness of breath and tingling in his fingers, arms, and face.

If a patient experiences *moderate anxiety*, you may note increased physiologic responses, alertness, and vigilance. His hearing may appear to be decreased because he's less able to respond to stimuli. He also may experience selective inattention, difficulty concentrating, and increased tension-relieving behav-

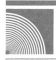

## When anxiety leads to aggression

What if your anxious patient becomes aggressive during your assessment? How should you handle the situation? By allowing him to express his feelings, so he can get them out of his system. Don't try to control or suppress his behavior. As you listen and talk, remember these points.

• Listen to the patient, but don't respond to provocative remarks or abusive language.

• Try not to show disapproval of his words or actions.

• Speak in short sentences. Avoid complex ideas or involved explanations.

• Use gestures and other nonverbal messages carefully. Smiling, nodding, and other positive messages may communicate the opposite of what you intend. The patient may misinterpret your smile and think you're laughing at him.

• Finally, try to remain relaxed. Don't appear aggressive or defensive.

iors, such as pacing, repetitive questioning, and shaking.

A patient with *severe anxiety* may exhibit the fight-or-flight survival response. In such a patient, epinephrine levels increase as do blood pressure, pulse rate, and respiratory rate. Vasoconstriction leads to pallor, and body temperature rises. Plus, the liver increases its glucose production.

This patient will also experience diaphoresis, dry mouth, urinary urgency, and decreased pain perception. He may be dazed or confused and unaware of what's going on around him, even when things are brought to his attention. His behavior may be automatic, aimed at reducing or relieving the anxiety. He

may complain of headache, nausea, dizziness, pounding heart, trembling, or hyperventilation. He also may indicate a sense of dread or impending doom. Severe anxiety can also distort the results of diagnostic tests, such as the plasma glucose, adrenal function, parathyroid hormone, and serum calcium tests.

If anxiety continues to escalate, the patient will develop signs of panic. The most severe form of anxiety, *panic-level anxiety* produces markedly disturbed behavior. Physiologic responses continue to increase, blood returns to major organs, blood pressure falls, motor coordination decreases, and the patient shows minimal response to pain, noise, and stimuli. He may shout, scream, act confused, or withdraw. (See *When anxiety leads to aggression*.)

### Emotional assessment

Emotional responses will vary from patient to patient. An anxious patient may feel apprehensive, nervous, irritable, frustrated, or confused. He may cry and withdraw from interactions with family and health care personnel. Or he may deny his anxiety. Such denial means that he won't be able to cope with the problem effectively.

*Family relationships.* Determine how the patient's current problems affect other family members. Understanding the family's structure, support system, and coping strategies can help you identify causes of stress, anxiety, and possible dysfunction within the family. How do other family members handle their anxiety? Does anxiety interfere with communication within the family? What resources do family members use to help them handle anxiety? As needed, help other family members deal with their anxiety so that they'll be able to provide emotional support for the patient. Also, help them to understand that some anxiety is a normal response to illness.

### Cognitive assessment
As you assess the patient, keep in mind that anxiety alters cognitive function. When a patient's anxiety increases, his perceptual field decreases, making him less responsive to environmental stimuli. Memory also decreases, making him unable to remember instructions or to follow simple directions. As well, altered thought processes decrease his ability to concentrate or solve problems.

*Role functions.* Assess how anxiety and altered cognitive function affect the patient's role functions. Do his current problems prevent him from meeting expectations in the family, at work, or in social settings? Has physical illness changed his usual roles?

### Spiritual assessment
Ask the patient about his belief system. Does he believe in a greater power? Does he feel he's acting according to his belief system, or is his anxiety interfering?

### Sources of anxiety
By identifying thoughts, activities, and situations that immediately precede or trigger anxiety, you can help the patient understand and cope with his problem. If he's extremely anxious, you may need to obtain this information from his family and friends or from other health care personnel. Then, after the patient's anxiety decreases, ask him to describe situations and interactions he thinks may be causing his anxiety.

### Coping mechanisms
Identify and explore the patient's past and present coping mechanisms. Are they adaptive or maladaptive? Adaptive coping mechanisms help the patient lower his anxiety and let him achieve goals in acceptable ways. These include seeking information, solving problems, and discussing the anxiety-producing situations with others.

Maladaptive coping mechanisms prevent the patient from handling anxiety effectively. Some examples include anger, denial, daydreaming, forgetfulness, depression, and excessive use of defense mechanisms.

# Immediate intervention

Immediate intervention can prevent moderate to severe anxiety from progressing to panic-level anxiety — an emergency situation. Interventions you may use include therapeutic communication to help the patient identify and deal with the cause of the anxiety, environmental manipulation, relaxation techniques, treatment for hyperventilation, and medication therapy.

### Therapeutic communication
To promote a trusting relationship with your patient, you need to show empathy, compassion, and objectivity. The best way to establish a therapeutic nurse-patient relationship is to project a calm, caring attitude. Active listening lets the patient know that his words and thoughts are important to you. Using therapeutic communication techniques helps you reduce the patient's anxiety — or at least prevent it from escalating.

If a patient has *mild to moderate*

*anxiety*, he'll still be able to solve problems, but if his anxiety increases, his ability to concentrate will diminish. You can help such a patient to identify the source of his anxiety by asking open-ended questions, clarifying his statements, and communicating your support.

If a patient has *severe to panic-level anxiety*, don't leave him alone. Staying with him decreases his sense of isolation and may enable you to protect him from physical danger.

**Identify sources of anxiety.** Using a matter-of-fact, nonjudgmental tone of voice, point out situations that seem to cause the patient anxiety. For example, you might say something such as "I notice that you've been talking more rapidly and perspiring more since your doctor came to see you. Did something upset you?" This helps make the patient aware of his behavior without making him defensive and more anxious.

**Explore sources of anxiety.** Using open-ended questions, gradually explore the apparent sources of the patient's anxiety. Initially, you may need to keep your comments brief because the patient may grow frustrated and more anxious as he becomes aware of what triggers his anxiety. If his anxiety does increase, redirect the conversation to earlier, more comfortable topics. Use positive reinforcement to increase his motivation to face the sources of his anxiety.

**Reinforce appropriate behavior.** Let the patient know when the anxiety he's experiencing is appropriate for the situation. For example, if the patient is waiting for test results to confirm a diagnosis, you might say something such as "It's hard to

wait, not knowing what the test results will be." Once he feels that you understand and care, he may be more comfortable talking about his concerns.

During the discussion, be alert to clues about specific causes of anxiety. For example, you may note that a misunderstanding about the test results is increasing his anxiety unnecessarily. Correct any misunderstandings and provide accurate information, if needed.

**Encourage realistic expectations.** Discuss the patient's expectations concerning his condition and treatment outcome. Reassure the patient, but be careful not to provide false hope. Avoid statements such as "Everything will be all right." Instead, say something such as "You seem upset. I'll stay with you and we can talk about what's upsetting you."

**Document anxiety episodes.** Note patterns of anxiety-related behaviors and adaptive coping strategies the patient uses. Also note which therapeutic techniques and care routines are most effective in relieving the patient's anxiety to ensure consistency in managing him.

### Environmental manipulation

Try to provide a quiet, soothing environment, free from excessive stimuli and potential hazards. Limit the patient's contact with others who are anxious, but allow enough contact with family and friends to avoid feelings of isolation or rejection.

Reduce the patient's anxiety by helping to meet his basic needs for warmth, food, fluids, elimination, pain relief, and social contact. Help him anticipate and avoid situations or people known to produce anxiety. As the patient's condition permits, provide an outlet for excess energy by suggesting such activities as walking, light exercise, painting, writing, or drawing.

## Relaxation techniques

Used to reduce anxiety, relaxation techniques can help patients who have the following problems: hypertension, dyspnea associated with chronic obstructive pulmonary disease, premature ventricular contractions, asthma, insomnia, stuttering, tension headaches, adverse effects of chemotherapy, ulcers, colitis, and pain associated with medical-surgical conditions or treatments. Commonly used techniques include deep breathing, abdominal breathing, progressive muscle relaxation, focused relaxation, and visualization.

*Deep breathing.* Perhaps the simplest and most frequently used relaxation technique, deep breathing involves having the patient inhale slowly through his mouth, then exhale slowly. With this technique, the patient redirects his attention, focusing on his control of a physiologic function. This, in turn, increases his feeling of overall control.

*Abdominal breathing.* Instruct the patient to sit or lie in a comfortable position, placing one hand on his lower abdomen. Have him slowly inhale while counting to four, hold the breath to the count of four, then exhale to the count of four. Tell him to repeat the process several times. Once he has established a regular breathing pattern, he can switch from counting to silently repeating a message — for example, ''I'm breathing in quiet, calm energy; as I exhale, I release tension and anxiety.''

*Progressive muscle relaxation.* Have

the patient alternately tense and relax muscle groups, noting the differences in the sensations of tension and relaxation. He should become more relaxed as he works through the major muscle groups of the body. This technique will also make him more aware of the signs of increasing muscular tension in everyday activities. (See *Using progressive muscle relaxation,* page 72.)

*Focused relaxation.* Help the patient assume a comfortable position in a quiet room with minimal distractions. Instruct him to empty his mind of all thoughts and to constantly repeat a chosen sound, word, or phrase while he focuses on his normal breathing rhythm. Tell him to dismiss immediately any distracting thoughts that might occur during the exercise.

*Visualization.* Have the patient sit or lie in a comfortable position in a quiet environment with his eyes closed. Then tell him to perform slow, rhythmic, deep breathing while relaxing tense portions of his body. At the same time, have him visualize a peaceful place where he would normally feel calm and relaxed. Or have him visualize himself successfully resolving the cause of his anxiety. After a specified time, tell the patient to count to four and open his eyes.

To reduce anxiety associated with pain, try this variation. First have the patient concentrate on the painful body part; then have him assign a visual symbol to the pain, such as a knot in the stomach. He can then imagine the knot relaxing and getting smaller.

## Treatment for hyperventilation

A patient who's hyperventilating requires immediate intervention to re-

## Using progressive muscle relaxation

To help your patient relieve anxiety, try progressive muscle relaxation (PMR). First, help him sit or lie in a comfortable position. Provide a cushion or pillow to support his head, as necessary.

Then have him slowly tense selected muscle groups for 5 to 7 seconds and relax them for 20 to 30 seconds. Tell him to focus on the different sensations of tension and relaxation. Have him repeat this pattern several times.

Typically, the patient should follow this sequence:
• hands, forearms, and biceps.
• head, neck, face, throat, and shoul-

ders. To avoid soft-tissue injury, caution him not to tighten his neck muscles excessively.
• chest, abdomen, and lower back. Tell him to avoid excessive tightening of back muscles.
• thighs, buttocks, legs, and feet.

If your patient's condition prevents him from tensing major muscle groups, try a modified form of PMR: Have your patient alternately tighten his jaw and relax it by letting it drop open slowly. Focusing on the jaw muscles can produce the same effect as tensing and relaxing major muscle groups.

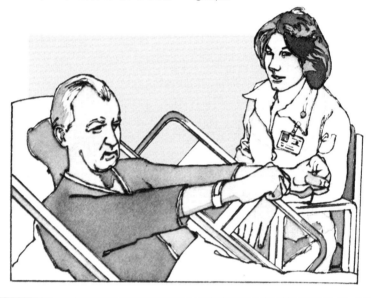

store the oxygen–carbon dioxide balance before he loses consciousness. Have the patient breathe into a paper bag or breathe with one nostril and his mouth closed. Reassure and calm him during the episode.

When he's breathing normally,

help him become more aware of his breathing patterns, so he can detect the beginning of rapid respirations that lead to hyperventilation. Then teach him breathing exercises, such as abdominal breathing, that will help him restore control and break the pattern of hyperventilation.

## Medication therapy

For short-term treatment, a patient with moderate to severe anxiety may benefit from an antianxiety drug, such as a benzodiazepine. A patient with severe to panic-level anxiety may need a tranquilizer before receiving an antianxiety drug. (See *Short-term medication therapy,* page 74.)

# Long-term management

A patient with chronic anxiety can benefit from long-term treatments, such as behavior modification, desensitization, medication therapy, and cognitive therapy. You may be involved in starting a patient on one or more of these therapies while he's hospitalized. But he will need to continue them after discharge.

## Behavior modification

With positive or negative reinforcement from others, an anxious patient can modify his behavior and learn new ways to cope with stress. Although the simplest behavioral technique is to reward positive behavior, negative reinforcement can be just as effective. For instance, a patient may learn to take his medication regularly because he has an uncomfortable physical experience when he doesn't. However, you should never use punishment to change behavior. The results tend to be short-lived and ultimately counterproductive.

*Social skills training.* A patient who feels anxious in social situations may benefit from special training to improve his social skills. In this form of behavior modification, the patient learns new social behaviors,

which he practices with a therapist and at appropriate times between sessions. The patient can then use these behaviors to improve communication and get along better with staff members as well as with family and friends who are trying to help him.

## Desensitization

Based on relaxation techniques, desensitization gradually makes the patient less vulnerable to the precipitating cause of his anxiety. This therapy is useful only when the patient's anxiety stems from a specific fear, such as a phobia.

In this progressive treatment, the patient first learns to attain muscle relaxation. While relaxed, he's gradually introduced to the cause of his anxiety — either in his imagination or in reality. For example, a patient with a phobic fear of elevators might imagine himself walking down a hallway toward an elevator. Then he imagines himself entering the elevator, pushing the elevator button, and so on, until he's able to visualize the entire sequence of activities necessary to complete an elevator ride while staying relaxed. A patient should practice this desensitization exercise twice a day until he can control his body's responses to tension. Then he's ready to use this technique with an actual elevator.

## Medication therapy

When anxiety interferes with a patient's ability to engage in a therapeutic relationship, extended medication therapy may be necessary. Make sure the patient understands the medication schedule, possible adverse effects, and drug interactions. Also, you need to advise him of any potential for addiction.

# Short-term medication therapy

Short-term drug therapy forms an important part of the treatment plan for some patients who suffer from anxiety.

### Commonly prescribed drugs
This list includes the most commonly prescribed antianxiety agents along with their recommended dosages.
• *alprazolam*: 0.25 to 0.5 mg P.O. t.i.d.
• *buspirone*: 5 to 10 mg P.O. t.i.d.
• *chlordiazepoxide*: 5 to 25 mg P.O. t.i.d. or q.i.d.
• *clorazepate*: 15 to 60 mg P.O. daily.
• *diazepam*: 2 to 10 mg P.O. b.i.d. to q.i.d.
• *halazepam*: 20 to 40 mg P.O. t.i.d. or q.i.d.
• *hydroxyzine*: 25 to 100 mg P.O. t.i.d. or q.i.d.
• *lorazepam*: 2 to 6 mg P.O. daily in divided doses
• *oxazepam*: 10 to 30 mg P.O. t.i.d. or q.i.d.
• *prazepam*: 20 to 40 mg P.O. daily in divided doses

### Nursing considerations
If a doctor prescribes one of these drugs for your patient, keep the following considerations in mind.
• If your patient is a pregnant woman, make sure her doctor knows of her condition.
• Instruct your patient to take the medication as prescribed and not to stop taking it abruptly.
• Monitor the patient's vital signs during the initial treatment.
• If your patient is also receiving another central nervous system (CNS) depressant or an anticholinergic, monitor him for additive effects, including drowsiness, a dry mouth, and constipation.
• Periodically monitor the patient's complete blood count and liver function.

• When reviewing laboratory studies, remember that antianxiety medications may cause increased levels of serum bilirubin; aspartate aminotransferase (AST), formerly SGOT; and alanine aminotransferase (ALT), formerly SGPT.
• If treatment with the antianxiety drug will continue after discharge, teach your patient to avoid alcohol and other CNS depressants, and to call his doctor before taking any over-the-counter medications.

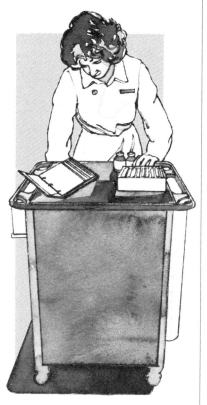

## Cognitive therapy

Such techniques as thought stopping and cognitive restructuring can help an anxious patient to adopt new thought patterns that support rational beliefs and appropriate behaviors.

***Thought stopping.*** Often used to treat obsessive-compulsive disorders and phobias, thought stopping helps the patient overcome disruptive thoughts. The technique is based on the premise that negative or frightening thoughts immediately precede similar emotions that can trigger negative behaviors.

To use this technique, instruct the patient to concentrate on the disruptive thought for a brief time, then consciously stop the thought and empty his mind. The patient can stop the thought by pinching himself, pressing his fingernails into his palm, clapping his hands loudly, or shouting "Stop!"

Tell your patient to practice thought stopping regularly over several days until he learns how to interrupt disruptive thoughts successfully. Then, instead of pinching himself or shouting when an unwanted thought intrudes, have him silently repeat a phrase such as "I don't need to think this thought. I can stop this thought and continue my normal activities."

***Cognitive restructuring.*** This approach involves changing the patient's attitudes, values, or beliefs through thought substitution, thought alteration, or problem solving.

*Thought substitution.* In this technique, the patient learns to replace negative thoughts with a positive assertion that's appropriate to the situation. He reinforces this asser-

tion with a series of positive thoughts until they replace the negative thoughts. For example, a patient who's waiting for a painful diagnostic test might tell himself, "This test will help the doctor determine how to treat my illness." He can build on this thought by adding, "I've handled other painful tests well."

For best results, use thought substitution when the patient's anxiety is mild. First, help the patient identify the negative thoughts he has as he goes about his daily activities. Some examples might include "I'll never get through this" or "I can never do anything right." Then help him identify a positive alternate statement, such as "I've survived lots of problems before" or "I'm really good at this."

Now have the patient write the positive statements on separate index cards and keep them nearby. Instruct him to read the top card several times a day until the positive thought replaces the negative one. Then he can move on to the statement on the next card. But encourage him not to switch to a new statement too quickly. Each statement must become familiar and easy to remember.

*Thought alteration.* Another approach to cognitive restructuring involves a six-step process for changing thoughts and actions. These steps include:
• recognizing irrational ideas that lead to anxiety
• gaining insight into the relationship between the ideas and anxiety
• analyzing thoughts objectively
• testing the validity of thoughts
• identifying assumptions that underlie the irrational ideas or thoughts
• changing the behavior patterns

that have resulted from irrational ideas and beliefs.

*Problem solving.* Cognitive restructuring also involves learning new ways to solve problems and respond to situations that trigger anxiety. This approach helps the patient accept that problems are a part of life and can be handled through systematic problem solving.

The steps involved in problem solving include:
• recognizing the presence of a situation that causes anxiety
• identifying the issues the situation presents
• developing alternative approaches to the problem
• reviewing possible consequences of each approach
• selecting an approach
• implementing the selected approach.

# Evaluation

As you care for your patient, you'll evaluate his behavior to determine his progress toward achieving treatment goals. Depending on the results of your evaluation, you may decide that a consultation with a psychiatrist or psychiatric clinical nurse specialist is necessary.

## Behavioral changes
During and after your interventions, evaluate any behavioral changes, noting the patient's ability to function. Focus on the following aspects: physical, emotional, cognitive, social, and spiritual.

*Physical function.* Can the patient meet his physical needs independently without undue anxiety? If

your interventions have been successful, any physical signs of anxiety you may observe should be mild.

*Emotional function.* Does the patient seem to have control over his emotions? After successful interventions, he won't report feelings of discomfort, fear, or dread, nor will he be angry, depressed, or agitated. Any anxiety he experiences should be mild, and it shouldn't interfere with his ability to perform necessary activities.

*Cognitive function.* Can the patient communicate clearly with others, recall information, and use appropriate techniques to manage anxiety? Can he discuss his problem-solving strategies? Have his judgment, insight, attention span, ability to concentrate, and decision-making skills improved?

*Social function.* Does the patient interact successfully with others? Does he communicate openly with family members and friends? Does he discuss his usual social activities comfortably?

*Spiritual needs.* Can the patient discuss his personal philosophy, values, and beliefs without undue anxiety? Does he seem hopeful?

## Requesting a consultation
Depending on the circumstances, you may request a consultation at any point in the nursing process. But typically, you'll assess, intervene, and evaluate the patient before consulting with a psychiatrist or psychiatric clinical nurse specialist. You should request a consultation in the following situations:
• The patient can't or won't talk about his anxiety.

• The patient's expressions of guilt and worthlessness indicate the potential for self-destructive behavior.
• The patient refuses treatment, resists nursing care, or engages in behaviors that are disruptive to other patients.
• Interventions to reduce severe anxiety don't decrease its physiologic signs.
• A patient with complex medical-surgical problems requires anti-anxiety medication.
• The patient requires follow-up or referral to a self-help group for anxiety-related problems.

## Suggested readings

Baumann, A., et al. *Decision Making in Psychiatric and Psychosocial Nursing.* Philadelphia: B.C. Decker, Inc., 1990.

Beck, C.K., et al. *Mental Health-Psychiatric Nursing: A Holistic Life-Cycle Approach*, 2nd ed. St. Louis: C.V. Mosby Co., 1988.

*Diagnostic and Statistical Manual of Mental Disorders,* 3rd ed., revised. Washington, D.C.: American Psychiatric Association, 1987.

Doenges, M.E., and Moorhouse, M.F. *Nurse's Pocket Guide: Nursing Diagnoses with Interventions,* 3rd ed. Philadelphia: F.A. Davis Co., 1990.

Halm, M.A. "Effects of Support Groups on Anxiety of Family Members During Critical Illness," *Heart & Lung* 19(1):62-71, January 1990.

Janosik, E.H., and Davies, J.L. *Psychiatric Mental Health Nursing*, 2nd ed. Boston: Jones & Bartlett Pubs., Inc., 1989.

Kniesl, C.R. "Combating Anxiety," *RN* 53(8):50-54, August 1990.

Pelletier, L.R., ed. *Psychiatric Nursing: Case Studies, Nursing Diagnoses, and Care Plans.* Springhouse, Pa.: Springhouse Corp., 1987.

Phipps, W.J., et al, eds. *Medical-Surgical Nursing: Concepts and Clinical Practice,* 3rd ed. St. Louis: C.V. Mosby Co., 1987.

Renfroe, K.L. "Effect of Progressive Relaxation on Dyspnea and State Anxiety in Patients with Chronic Obstructive Pulmonary Disease," *Heart & Lung* 17(4):408-13, July 1988.

Sparks, S.M., and Taylor, C.M. *Nursing Diagnosis Reference Manual.* Springhouse, Pa.: Springhouse Corp., 1991.

Stuart, G.W., and Sundeen, S.J. *Pocket Nurse Guide to Psychiatric Nursing.* St. Louis: C.V. Mosby Co., 1988.

Titlebaum, H.M. "Relaxation," *Holistic Nursing Practice* (3):17-25, May 1988.

# 5

# CONFUSION

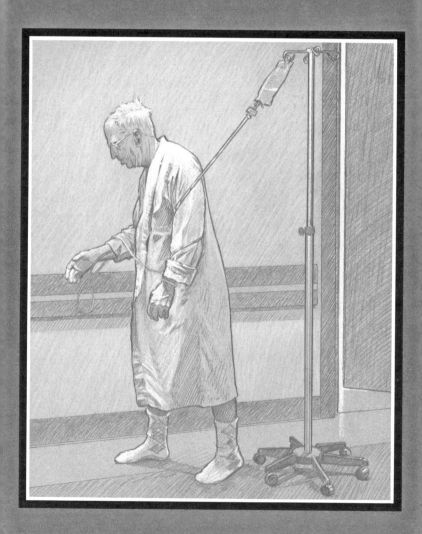

When you think of a confused patient, you probably picture an elderly person with Alzheimer's disease. But confusion may result from several other causes, and it may develop at any age.

Confusion arises from an impairment of the areas of the brain that control such higher functions as comprehension, abstract thinking, judgment, reasoning, attention, and memory. When confusion results from a reversible condition and progresses rapidly, it's called *delirium*. When confusion results from a chronic cerebral nerve disruption and progresses slowly, it's called *dementia*. A patient can suffer from delirium and dementia at the same time.

### Causes of delirium

Delirium may result from systemic problems, such as infection, oxygen deprivation, acid-base imbalance, drug toxicity or interactions, or a reaction to a drug. Hospitalized patients under extreme stress may experience delirium from a combination of factors — for instance, sleep deprivation, use of sedatives or analgesics, metabolic fluctuations, and overstimulation. (See *Identifying causes of delirium.*)

### Causes of dementia

Dementia may result from irreversible disorders, including neurologic disorders such as Alzheimer's and Huntington's disease as well as acquired immunodeficiency syndrome (AIDS). It may also result from treatable causes, such as Parkinson's disease, normal pressure hydrocephalus, myocardial infarction, central nervous system (CNS) infections, brain tumors, and metabolic disorders. (See *Identifying treatable causes of dementia,* page 80.)

CHECKLIST

## Identifying causes of delirium

Delirium may result from the following potentially reversible systemic problems:

☐ *Acid-base imbalance* — acidosis, alkalosis

☐ *Body-temperature changes* — hyperthermia, hypothermia

☐ *Cardiovascular dysfunction* — acute myocardial infarction, arrhythmias, cerebrovascular accident (delirium occurs afterward), congestive heart failure, disseminated intravascular coagulation, hypovolemia

☐ *Central nervous system (CNS) dysfunction* — CNS infection or inflammation, head trauma, seizures (delirium occurs afterward)

☐ *Drug toxicity* — alcohol, amphetamines, antiarrhythmics, anticonvulsants, antidepressants, antihistamines, barbiturates, beta blockers, cocaine, corticosteroids, digitalis, diuretics, lithium, monoamine oxidase inhibitors, opioids, penicillins, phenothiazines

☐ *Electrolyte imbalances* — hypercalcemia, hypermagnesemia, hypomagnesemia, hypernatremia, hyponatremia

☐ *Endocrine dysfunction* — adrenal, parathyroid, pituitary, thyroid

☐ *Hepatic dysfunction* — liver failure

☐ *Infection* — sepsis

☐ *Oxygen deprivation* — anemia, hypoventilation

☐ *Poisoning* — cyanide, heavy metals

☐ *Renal dysfunction* — kidney failure

☐ *Vitamin deficiencies* — folic acid, niacin, thiamine, vitamin B.

Although about 10% to 20% of dementia cases are reversible, the disorder is frequently misdiagnosed as irreversible dementia. Thus, many patients don't receive proper care. Depression also may be mistaken for dementia in elderly patients because the signs and symptoms are similar — forgetful-

CHECKLIST

### Identifying treatable causes of dementia

When dementia results from the following causes, it can often be successfully treated:
☐ *Cardiovascular dysfunction*—arrhythmias, cerebrovascular accident, congestive heart failure, myocardial infarction, subdural hematoma
☐ *Depression*
☐ *Drug toxicity*—alcohol, barbiturates, digitalis, diuretics, methyldopa, oral antidiabetics, phenothiazines, propranolol, tranquilizers
☐ *Electrolyte imbalances*—hypernatremia, hyponatremia, hypercalcemia
☐ *Endocrine dysfunction*—Addison's disease, Cushing's syndrome, diabetes mellitus, hypoglycemia, hypothyroidism
☐ *Hepatic dysfunction*—cirrhosis, hepatitis, Wilson's disease
☐ *Infection*
☐ *Neuromuscular dysfunction*—Parkinson's disease
☐ *Normal pressure hydrocephalus*
☐ *Poisoning*—bromide, carbon monoxide, lead, mercury
☐ *Pulmonary dysfunction*—chronic obstructive pulmonary disease, pulmonary emboli
☐ *Renal dysfunction*—dehydration, urinary tract infection that exacerbates mild nephritis
☐ *Toxic metabolic disorders*—pernicious anemia
☐ *Tumor*
☐ *Vitamin deficiencies*—ascorbic acid, folic acid, niacin, riboflavin, thiamine, vitamin $A_1$, vitamin $B_{12}$.

ness, withdrawal, and diminished ability to think. If a patient has symptoms of both dementia and depression, the depression should be treated first. If the dementia stemmed from the depression, the symptoms of dementia will also disappear.

# Assessment

Because many of the signs and symptoms are similar, delirium and dementia may be difficult to distinguish. But thorough nursing and medical assessments can lead to an accurate diagnosis.

Your assessment of a confused patient consists of a health history, a mental status evaluation, and a physical examination. Typically, the patient's doctor will order diagnostic tests to determine if the cause of confusion is treatable. (See *Criteria for diagnosing delirium and dementia,* opposite, and *Comparing delirium and dementia,* page 82.)

### Health history

Certain cognitive and sensory deficits may make effective communication difficult or impossible for a confused patient. For example, memory loss and disorientation may undermine his ability to understand your questions and answer them accurately, and speech deficits may slow the process of gathering information. Having a family member or close friend present may help you obtain an accurate history. When this isn't possible, you may be able to overcome some communication barriers by spending extra time with the patient.

Note the patient's symptoms and determine when they began. Keep in mind that a person with dementia usually becomes disoriented first to time, then to place and person. To prevent embarrassment, a patient may fabricate events. He may also be restless and agitated and exhibit a deterioration in social skills. If he becomes extremely restless, you can shorten your interview or finish it

# Criteria for diagnosing delirium and dementia

How does a doctor distinguish delirium from dementia? Typically, he'll rely on the criteria spelled out in the *Diagnostic and Statistical Manual of Mental Disorders,* 3rd edition (revised).

**Delirium**
The criteria for diagnosing delirium include:
• diminished attention span
• disorganized thinking
• at least two of the following:
– decreased level of consciousness
– misinterpretations, illusions, hallucinations, or other perceptual problems
– sleep-wake cycle disruptions with insomnia or daytime drowsiness
– enhanced or diminished psychomotor activity
– disorientation to time, place, or person
– loss of short- or long-term memory
• signs and symptoms that appear over hours or days and usually fluctuate as the day progresses
• evidence of an organic cause of the delirium discovered during the history, physical examination, or laboratory tests. (Without such evidence, an organic cause can be assumed if the delirium can't be traced to any nonorganic mental disorder.)

**Dementia**
The criteria for diagnosing dementia include:
• impaired short-term and long-term memory
• at least two of the following:
– decreased abstract thinking
– faulty judgment
– other problems of higher cortical function, such as aphasia, apraxia, and constructional difficulty (an inability to copy three-dimensional figures or to arrange blocks or sticks into patterns)
– personality changes, such as exaggeration of certain traits
• severe problems with work, social

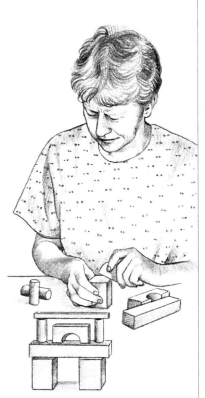

activities, and interpersonal relationships
• confusion that remains after delirium has been treated
• evidence of a distinct organic cause of the dementia discovered during the history, physical examination, or laboratory tests. (Without such evidence, an organic cause can be assumed if the dementia can't be traced to any nonorganic mental problem.)

## Comparing delirium and dementia

| ONSET AND DURATION | CAUSES | SIGNS AND SYMPTOMS |
| --- | --- | --- |
| **Delirium** | | |
| • Sudden onset; may affect any age-group<br>• Typically lasts only 1 month or less | Hyperthermia, infection, sensory deprivation or overload, space-occupying lesions, toxins, trauma | Agitation, confusion, diffuse disorganized thoughts, slowed EEG activity, emotional instability, hallucinations, illusions, impaired decision making, lack of inhibitions, restlessness |
| **Dementia** | | |
| • Gradual onset; typically affects persons age 65 and older<br>• Progressive and long-term; may be halted or reversed occasionally | Anemia, brain tissue atrophy, encephalitis, HIV-related disorders, hyper- or hypotension, hyper- or hypothermia, hypoglycemia, meningitis, normal pressure hydrocephalus, toxins, tumors, vitamin deficiencies | Agitation, confusion, diminished attention span, emotional lability, impaired judgment, memory loss, resistance to change, restlessness |

when he has calmed down.

Ask about past and present illnesses and any incidents of head trauma. Determine which prescription and over-the-counter drugs the patient is taking; they may be causing his confusion—especially if he's taking several together. To determine his nutritional status ask about his diet. Find out who prepares his food and when he last ate.

Next, find out whether the patient drinks alcohol. If so, how much? In an alcoholic, confusion may begin anywhere from 24 hours to 10 days after the last drink. Ask too about illicit drugs. When did he last use such drugs? Acute withdrawal from barbiturates and certain illicit drugs may cause confusion and other changes in intellectual function.

Ask if the patient or any family members have a history of mental illness, especially depression. Also, find out if the patient has experi-

enced any acute or long-term stress. Such stress may result from the death of a close friend or family member, sleep deprivation, a change in job status, and a loss of income—to name just a few causes. AIDS patients are especially vulnerable to confusion from stress. The lack of social supports, the stigma of the disease, and, in some cases, the death of friends from AIDS can lead to panic-level anxiety, which in turn can cause confusion.

### Mental status evaluation

Next, assess the patient's mental status to help determine whether his confusion results from delirium or dementia. Suspect delirium if you note disorientation to time, place, and person; a disturbed sleep-wake cycle; clouding of consciousness; visual hallucinations; illusions; delusions; agitation; and impaired attention, concentration, and memory.

Suspect dementia if the onset of confusion is insidious. Typically, it begins with the patient forgetting recent events. Or he may forget how to perform simple tasks. Other early signs include difficulty learning and remembering new information, a deterioration in personal hygiene and appearance, and an inability to concentrate. As the disease progresses, tasks requiring abstract thinking and activities requiring judgment become more difficult, and long-term memory loss occurs. Eventually, the patient has trouble carrying out voluntary movements (apraxia), speaking (aphasia), and recognizing objects (agnosia). He may also have hallucinations and periods of agitation.

*Memory loss.* To assess short-term memory loss, show the patient three unrelated objects. Five minutes later, ask him to recall them.

To assess long-term memory loss, ask the patient to recall past events (for instance, what he had for dinner the night before) or common facts (for instance, the name of the President). Or you can quiz him about personal information, such as his date of birth, birthplace, or occupation. To determine the extent of cognitive impairment, use Goldfarb's 10-point scale (see *Evaluating cognitive impairment,* page 84).

*Judgment and abstract thinking.* To evaluate judgment, ask the patient or a family member how the patient handles various interpersonal, family, financial, or occupational issues. Evaluate his behavior to see if his social judgment is impaired. For instance, ask the patient what he would do if he were in a crowded theater and smelled smoke. Or ask his family if he has ever become violent or if he wears clothing inappropriate to the season. Check the patient's abstract thinking by seeing if he can find similarities between words or concepts. For example, when you ask him if apples and bananas have anything in common, can he tell you that they're both fruits?

### Physical examination

To help determine the organic cause of the patient's confusion, you may perform a complete physical examination. As you do, be alert for the following clues: lacerations or contusions, central or peripheral cyanosis (hypoxemia), fever, and increased heart and respiratory rates.

### Diagnostic testing

The patient's doctor may order certain diagnostic tests to determine the cause of the confusion. Routine studies, such as a complete blood count, electrolyte levels, blood urea nitrogen levels, arterial blood gas studies, urinalysis, and an electrocardiogram, can all help pinpoint an underlying physiologic cause. A computed tomography scan and a magnetic resonance imaging scan can detect focal lesions, such as tumors and intracerebral hematomas. And an EEG will detect abnormal brain electrical activity. In some cases, invasive procedures also may be performed. For example, if the doctor suspects meningitis, he may perform a lumbar puncture to help diagnose a CNS infection. (See *Using diagnostic tests,* page 85.)

---

# Intervention

Your goals and interventions will vary, depending on whether your patient's confusion results from de-

## Evaluating cognitive impairment

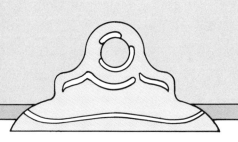

To determine your patient's level of cognitive impairment, try using Goldfarb's 10-point scale. First, ask the patient the following questions:

| ✔ | 1. Where are we right now? |
|---|---|
|   | 2. What's the location of this place? |
| ✔ | 3. What month is it? |
| ✔ | 4. What day of the week or month is it? |
| ✔ | 5. What year is it? |
|   | 6. How old are you? |
| ✔ | 7. When were you born? |
| ✔ | 8. Where were you born? |
|   | 9. Who is the current President of the United States? |
|   | 10. Who was the President before him? |

Now, count the number of incorrect responses and determine the level of impairment by using this scale:
• 0 to 2 incorrect answers—no impairment or mild impairment
• 3 to 8 incorrect answers—moderate impairment
• 9 to 10 incorrect answers—severe impairment

## Using diagnostic tests

A doctor may order these tests to detect the cause of a patient's confusion.

| TEST | POSSIBLE CAUSE |
|------|----------------|
| Arterial blood gases | Hypoxemia |
| AST, ALT, and serum bilirubin | Hepatic encephalopathy |
| Chest X-ray | Pulmonary disease |
| Complete blood count | Anemia |
| EEG | Cerebral ischemia and hypoxia, possibly caused by cardiac insufficiency |
| Serum $B_{12}$, folic acid, and thiamine | Vitamin deficiency |
| Serum calcium and phosphate | Parathyroid disease |
| Serum creatinine and blood urea nitrogen | Renal encephalopathy |
| Serum glucose | Hypoglycemia |
| Serum thyroxine and serum free thyroxine | Thyroid disease |
| Sodium and potassium | Adrenal disease |
| Urinalysis | Urinary tract infection |
| Veneral Disease Research Laboratory slide test | Syphilis |

lirium or dementia. Your goal is to return a delirious patient to his state of health before the onset of confusion. For a patient with dementia, your goal is to maintain his present level of functioning. If the patient has progressive dementia, your goal is to improve his quality of life.

Your interventions may include using therapeutic communication, controlling the environment, promoting independence, providing comfort measures, administering drug therapy, and supporting the patient's family.

### Therapeutic communication

A confused patient has an impaired ability to think, reason, understand language, and perceive his environment, so you'll have to make a special effort to communicate with him. Begin each conversation by addressing the patient by name and identifying yourself. Speak calmly and slowly in a normal tone of voice, use simple words and sentences, and try to sound and look nonthreatening. Stand directly in his line of vision and maintain eye contact. Ask one question at a time and give the patient time to answer. Try to keep him focused on the topic under discussion. Move slowly, don't overreact, and be aware of your own emotional responses to the patient.

If the patient has a hearing impairment, you may need to repeat yourself, but be aware that constant repetition can be frustrating for both of you. If the patient uses a hearing aid, make sure that it's working. If he has a vision problem, make sure that he's wearing his glasses or contact lenses so he doesn't misinterpret your actions.

### Environmental manipulation
Assess the patient's hospital room to ensure that the environment is neither over- nor understimulating. Either condition can exacerbate confusion. For example, lights can cause distortions and shadows that may frighten the patient. As necessary, rearrange lamps and change light bulbs for a more relaxing environment. Also, keep the drapes open to let in natural light and help orient the patient to the time of day. A clock, a calendar, and familiar objects from home are also helpful. If necessary, reorient the patient whenever you begin a conversation.

Also, make sure the patient's environment is safe. Ensure that the lighting is adequate to help prevent the patient from tripping. Keep the bed in the lowest position and the side rails up. And check on the patient frequently.

Because the confused patient has difficulty coping with change, try to establish a predictable routine and provide continuity of care. Schedule such activities as washing, dressing, and eating at the same time each day to help decrease the patient's fear and frustration. When possible, advise him of upcoming treatments and procedures.

### Independence for the patient
Whenever possible, allow the patient to make decisions about his care. For instance, you might allow the patient to choose whether he wants his bath in the morning or evening. This can help the patient maintain a sense of control over his life.

### Comfort measures
Using comfort measures, such as repositioning and massage, can help reduce a confused patient's agitation. Begin by determining the source of the patient's agitation. Then try to alleviate it. For instance, a patient may be restless because he needs to go to the bathroom or is in pain. Or he may be agitated during or after a family visit. Hemodynamic changes can also cause agitation and increase confusion. So can diseases that cause hypoxemia, such as pneumonia. Plus, certain medications can cause agitation.

In some cases, you may need to use restraints to protect a confused patient from harming himself and others. Soft restraints are generally effective, but in some cases — particularly with patients who are withdrawing from illicit drugs — leather restraints may be necessary. Remember, use restraints only as a last alternative. Before applying them, check your hospital policy.

### Drug therapy
Depending on the cause of confusion, the patient's doctor may order medications to control the symptoms or to treat an underlying disorder, such as depression.

Drug therapy shouldn't be used for any patient who's in shock or a coma or who has unstable vital signs. If a patient's confusion results from drug or alcohol abuse, he'll need to begin a detoxification program. The doctor may order medications to reduce the severity of withdrawal syndrome and, if appropriate, to reduce the risk of life-threatening withdrawal reactions.

Depending on the situation, the doctor may prescribe a neuroleptic, an antianxiety agent, or a beta blocker.

*Neuroleptics.* Neuroleptic (or antipsychotic) medications change the mood and thoughts of a patient who has an altered perception of reality. Although their exact mechanism of action is unclear, these major tranquilizers can diminish agitation, disorganized thinking, and withdrawn behavior. Neuroleptics include phenothiazines, such as chlorpromazine (Thorazine), and nonphenothiazines, such as haloperidol (Haldol).

*Antianxiety agents.* These drugs (also known as benzodiazepines) are minor tranquilizers. They induce mild sedation and reduce anxiety and tension.

*Beta blockers.* This group of drugs, which includes propranolol (Inderal), may help treat agitation and anxiety when other drugs don't work. Keep in mind that beta blockers can cause orthostatic hypotension, increasing the risk of falls; you'll need to closely monitor the blood pressure of a patient receiving one of these drugs. Also, you must use beta blockers cautiously in patients who have cardiac or pulmonary disease.

### Support for the family
Don't forget that a confused patient's family members also need teaching and support — especially if the patient has progressive dementia. Because of the overwhelming, long-term demands of caring for such a patient, families are at high risk for developing depression and other stress-related illnesses. So encourage them to discuss their feelings with you, and help them find home care or social-service agencies

## Coping with a confused patient

Caring for a confused patient can make you feel overwhelmed and depressed. Such a patient can be frustrating, exhausting, and even frightening if he's violent.

To reduce the stress of caring for a confused patient, share your feelings with other nurses and ask them to share ideas on how to best handle him. You might also consult a psychiatric clinical nurse specialist to find new alternatives for dealing with your patient.

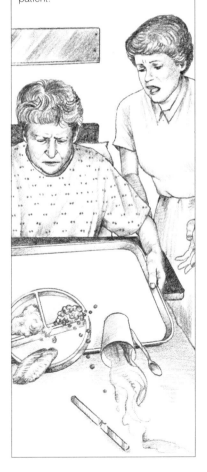

### Determining the severity of dementia

When you assess a patient with dementia, you can use these broad guidelines to determine whether the problem is mild, moderate, or severe.
• *Mild dementia:* The patient's work and social activities are significantly affected, but he can still live independently and maintain personal hygiene. His judgment is basically intact.
• *Moderate dementia:* Independent living is dangerous, and the patient requires some supervision.
• *Severe dementia:* The patient needs constant supervision to carry out activities of daily living. He can't maintain even minimal personal hygiene and may be incoherent or mute.

that can provide relief. Also refer them to an appropriate support group. (See *Coping with a confused patient,* page 87.)

# Evaluation

Make sure you've developed reasonable goals to help the patient and his family cope with his condition. For instance, your goal for a patient with debilitating dementia might be to decrease his agitation. For a patient with drug-induced delirium, you might have a short-term goal of decreasing assaultive episodes and a long-term goal of returning to normal cognitive functioning. Then be realistic when evaluating the patient's progress.

A patient with physiologically induced delirium should return to normal once the underlying disease has been treated, unless he has suffered permanent damage. Your interventions should help a patient with progressive dementia function to the best of his ability. This patient will need frequent reevaluation and follow-up care because his ability to function will progressively deteriorate. (See *Determining the severity of dementia.*)

### Requesting a consultation
Depending on the circumstances, you may request a consultation at any point in the nursing process. Typically, you'll assess, intervene, and evaluate the patient before consulting with a psychiatrist or psychiatric clinical nurse specialist.

Sometimes, though, you'll request a consultation earlier. For instance, you should seek a psychiatric consultation if a previously oriented, sociable patient suddenly becomes confused or agitated, or loses his memory, and a physiologic cause is ruled out. Also ask for a psychiatric consultation if a patient talks about dying, says he wants to die, starts giving away personal belongings, or becomes increasingly withdrawn.

### Suggested readings

Baker, F. "Screening Tests for Cognitive Impairment," *Hospital and Community Psychiatry* 40(4):339-40, April 1989.
Balster, G., et al. "Cognitive Impairment among Geropsychiatric Outpatients," *Hospital and Community Psychiatry* 41(5):556-58, May 1990.
Besdine, R. "Dementia and Delirium," in *Geriatric Medicine,* 2nd ed. Edited by Rowe, J., and Besdine, R. Boston: Little, Brown & Co., 1988.
Cohen, G. "Alzheimer's Disease: Clinical Update," *Hospital and Community Psychiatry* 41(5):496-97, May 1990.
Curl, A. "Agitation and the Older Adult," *Journal of Psychosocial Nursing and*

*Mental Health Services* 27(12):12-14, December 1989.

*Diagnostic and Statistical Manual of Mental Disorders,* 3rd ed., revised. Washington, D.C.: American Psychiatric Association, 1987.

Duffey, B.D. "Demented, Old, and Alone," *American Journal of Nursing* 89(2):212-16, February 1989.

Farran, C.J., and Keane-Hagerty, E. "Communicating Effectively with Dementia Patients," *Journal of Psychosocial Nursing and Mental Health Services* 27(5):13-16, 31-32, May 1989.

Gomez, G., and Gomez, E. "Delirium," *Geriatric Nursing* 8(6):330-32, November-December 1987.

Haggerty, J., et al. "Differential Diagnosis of Pseudodementia in the Elderly," *Geriatrics* 43(3):61-74, March 1988.

Harvis, K.A., and Rabins, P.V. "Dementia: Helping Family Caregivers Cope," *Journal of Psychosocial Nursing and Mental Health Services* 27(5):6-8, 10-12, 31-32, May 1989.

Lentz, J. "Therapy with Clients with Organic Mental Disorders," in *Mental Health-Psychiatric Nursing: A Holistic Life-Cycle Approach,* 2nd ed. Edited by Beck, C.K., et al. St. Louis: C.V. Mosby Co., 1988.

Matzo, M. "Confusion in Older Adults: Assessment and Differential Diagnosis," *Nurse Practitioner* 15(9):32-36, September 1990.

Rockwood, K. "Acute Confusion in Elderly Medical Patients," *Journal of the American Geriatrics Society* 37(2):150-54, February 1989.

Ronsman, K. "Pseudodementia...False Confusion," *Geriatric Nursing* 9(1):50-52, January-February 1988.

Salzman, C. "Treatment of the Agitated Demented Elderly Patient," *Hospital and Community Psychiatry* 39(11):1143-44, November 1988.

Stewart, J. "Diagnosing and Treating Depression in the Hospitalized Elderly," *Geriatrics* 46(1):64-72, January 1991.

Strumpf, N., et al. "Restraint-free Care: From Dream to Reality," *Geriatric Nursing* 11(3):122-24, May-June 1990.

Swanson, B., et al. "Dementia and Depression in Persons with AIDS: Causes and Care," *Journal of Psychosocial Nursing and Mental Health Services* 28(10):33-41, October 1990.

Teri, L., et al. "Cognitive Deterioration in Alzheimer's Disease: Behavioral and Health Factors," *Journal of Gerontology* 45(2):58-63, March 1990.

Wilson, H.S., and Kneisl, C.R. *Psychiatric Nursing,* 3rd ed. Menlo Park, Calif.: Addison-Wesley Publishing Co., 1988.

# 6

# DEPRESSION

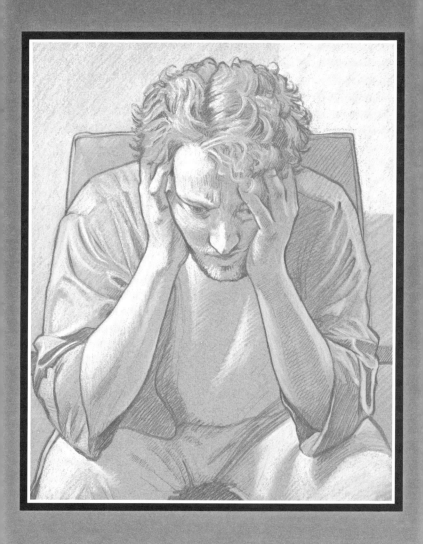

Most people experience transient feelings of sadness, dejection, or unhappiness. And you can certainly expect hospital patients to have such periodic bouts of "the blues" because of their unfamiliar and unsettled situation.

But when these common emotions become more intense and last longer than usual, your patient may be suffering from depression. In such cases, you'll observe disrupted thought processes, impaired communication, and sensory dysfunction. And you'll need to intervene effectively to help your patient avoid the serious — possibly even life-threatening — effects of depression.

This chapter begins with an overview of the types of depression, then covers the risk groups and the possible underlying causes. Next comes a section on how to assess a patient for depression. Then you'll review how to intervene to help a depressed patient. The final section of the chapter discusses evaluating the success of your interventions.

# Understanding depression

Depression has been defined as an emotional reaction, an altered mood state, and a physical symptom complex accompanied by a negative self-concept, low self-esteem, and regressive or self-punitive thoughts or behavior. It differs from grief (which is associated with a specific loss or separation), occurs in predictable phases, and tends to be self-limiting.

## Types of depression
Depression may be internal or reactive. *Internal depression* results

when a person experiences emotional turmoil. This primary depression has no known outside cause. *Reactive depression is secondary to* a change in a patient's environment, life situation, or general condition. In a hospitalized patient, you may see this type of depression occur in response to an illness or a change in physiologic condition or as a reaction to a medication.

The types of depression include mild depression, major depression, melancholia, dysthymia, seasonal affective disorder, manic-depressive illness (bipolar disorder), and cyclothymia.

*Mild depression.* Illness and the effects of hospitalization commonly produce mild depression among patients — especially those who feel unusually discouraged or desperate. For instance, a terminally ill patient will experience mild depression during the grieving process. Such a patient may be quiet, withdrawn, and melancholy before he gradually accepts reality.

Keep in mind that mild depression can produce serious medical consequences. Research has shown that it raises the rate of complications in patients with coronary artery disease, increasing the risk of myocardial infarction, surgery, and death.

*Major depression.* A person who's depressed or takes no pleasure in daily activities over a 2-week period may be experiencing a major depressive episode. Major depression can be diagnosed only after organic causes, schizophrenia, and other psychotic disorders are ruled out. (See *Criteria for diagnosing major depression,* page 92.)

A patient with major depression can't concentrate or make decisions, which may impair his ability to

## Criteria for diagnosing major depression

A doctor can diagnose a major depressive episode only after ruling out organic causes, schizophrenia, and other psychotic disorders. According to the *Diagnostic and Statistical Manual of Mental Disorders*, 3rd edition (revised), a doctor can diagnose such an episode when a patient experiences a depressed mood or a loss of interest in pleasure and at least four of the following symptoms in a 2-week period:
• a significant weight loss or weight gain without dieting, an increased or decreased appetite or, in children, a failure to achieve expected weight increases
• insomnia or hypersomnia
• psychomotor agitation or retardation
• fatigue or listlessness
• feelings of worthlessness or guilt
• reduced ability to think, concentrate, or make decisions
• recurrent thoughts of death or suicidal ideation.

function in social settings or at work. He also may have delusional thoughts, feel guilty and inadequate, and have persistent thoughts of disease, death, nihilism, persecution, or a need for punishment.

**Melancholia.** Similar to major depression, melancholia produces symptoms that are more or less constant over a prolonged period. A melancholic patient may feel apathetic and fail to react to pleasurable stimuli. Regularly depressed, the patient may wake up 2 hours earlier than usual and feel worse in the morning. He also may experience a sudden, significant weight gain or loss as well as psychomotor retardation or agitation. Other char-

acteristics include one or more previous major depressive episodes followed by complete, or nearly complete, recovery; no significant personality disturbances before the first major depressive episode; and a previous positive response to antidepressant therapy.

**Dysthymia.** Also known as depressive neurosis, dysthymia is characterized by a chronic depressive mood that's more or less constant for 1 year in children and 2 years in adults. Typical symptoms are similar to those of major depression. However, the dysthymic patient displays only two symptoms of major depression, and he doesn't have delusional thoughts. Dysthymia is especially common among patients with a history of anorexia, substance abuse, anxiety disorders, or rheumatoid arthritis. The diagnosis doesn't apply to patients taking medications known to cause depression as an adverse reaction.

**Seasonal affective disorder.** A patient with this disorder regularly becomes depressed and reclusive during the fall and winter. Typically, symptoms become most severe during January and February.
    Seasonal affective disorder isn't usually diagnosed in women until they reach their early 40s, although they may have a history of symptoms since their 20s. The disorder can be diagnosed only after symptoms occur in 3 years — 2 of which must be consecutive.

**Manic-depressive illness.** The most common mental disorder, manic-depressive illness affects between 1% and 5% of all adults, striking men and women equally. This disorder is characterized by abrupt mood swings from depression to elation (mania) or by prolonged episodes of either mood. In fact, severe depression may last for weeks. During periods of elation, the patient may be extremely talkative, jovial, and energetic. The manic patient may have an exaggerated sense of self-worth, may appear hyperactive and irritable, and may not require sleep for days. He also may lack judgment and insight into his behavior, become hypersexual, shop compulsively, or make careless financial decisions.

Before establishing a diagnosis of manic-depressive illness, the doctor must rule out organic conditions, schizophrenia, and other psychotic disorders. (See *Criteria for diagnosing a manic episode,* page 94.)

*Cyclothymia.* In this disorder, moderate depression alternates with moderate mania. This form of depression usually begins in late adolescence or early adulthood and persists for at least 2 years. Unlike manic-depressive illness, cyclothymia rarely affects the person's ability to function in social settings or at work. However, some patients do have difficulty maintaining personal relationships and performing at school or work.

## Who's at risk
According to the American Psychiatric Association, 10% of men and 26% of women in the United States will suffer from clinical depression at some point in their lives. About 3% of these men and 6% of these women will need to be hospitalized for their depression. The workdays lost, the staggering hospital costs, and the personal toll on family and friends compound the problem.

Although depression can strike a person of any age, the first symptoms commonly occur in those be-

tween the ages of 20 and 24. Persons with a family history of depression are three times more likely to develop depression themselves. Other risk factors include low family income, unemployment, obesity, normal hormonal fluctuations, and lack of confidence.

The risk groups include married women, children and adolescents, older adults, dysfunctional families, bereaved persons, hospitalized patients, myocardial infarction (MI) patients, acquired immunodeficiency syndrome (AIDS) patients, cancer patients, demented patients, schizophrenic patients, and caregivers of patients with chronic disorders.

*Married women.* The classic profile of a person at risk is a married woman with low self-esteem and three or more children at home. Women who've lost their mothers before age 11 are also prone to depression.

*Children and adolescents.* Children experience depression with symptoms similar to those of adults. During adolescence, additional symptoms may include sulking, withdrawal, and restlessness — all of which may be misdiagnosed as part of the normal maturing process.

*Older adults.* As many as 25% of older adults who live in institutions experience depression. In many cases, the symptoms are mistakenly considered part of the normal aging process or attributed to medical conditions.

*Dysfunctional families.* Depressed people tend to come from families that are emotionally unhealthy. Specifically, these dysfunctional families don't communicate or solve problems well.

## Criteria for diagnosing a manic episode

In manic-depressive illness, periods of depression alternate with periods of elation (mania). During the manic period, the patient's mood is abnormally elevated, expansive, or irritable. Also, according to the criteria spelled out in the *Diagnostic and Statistical Manual of Mental Disorders*, 3rd edition (revised), the patient will experience at least three of the following symptoms (four, if his mood is only irritable):
• inflated self-esteem or sense of self-worth
• reduced need for sleep
• verbosity
• flights of ideas or a feeling that thoughts are racing
• poor concentration
• increase in goal-directed actions or psychomotor agitation
• excessive involvement in pleasurable activities that have a high risk of a negative outcome — buying sprees, for example.

If the patient is experiencing *manic syndrome,* his mood disturbance will be severe enough to impair his ability to function in social settings or at work. He may require hospitalization to prevent harming himself or others. This type of impairment doesn't occur in a patient experiencing *hypomanic syndrome.*

Delusions and hallucinations rule out a diagnosis of manic-depressive illness. This diagnosis also doesn't apply to patients whose depression stems from an organic disorder, schizophrenia, schizophreniform disorder, delusional disorder, or an unspecified psychotic disorder.

**Bereaved persons.** Bereavement, a normal life process, may progress to depression when a person doesn't have the resources to overcome an actual or potential loss. A pathologic exaggeration of grief, depression affects the person's daily life for a prolonged period, usually a year or more.

**Hospitalized patients.** Between 40% and 60% of hospitalized patients experience depression — compared with 20% of those treated as outpatients. In a hospitalized patient, you may observe such signs of depression as a failure to comply with treatments or nursing interventions, a lack of motivation, or denial of the medical diagnosis. Depression is especially likely to strike the patient whose ability to function has decreased, such as the patient who has lost the use of a limb or who has suffered an amputation.

**MI patients.** About 45% of patients experience depression following an MI. This depression may result from diminished self-esteem and a feeling of powerlessness. Post-MI depression is often difficult to diagnose because the effects of an MI — such as decreased appetite and weight loss — are similar to the signs and symptoms of depression.

**AIDS patients.** Depression, commonly misdiagnosed as dementia, occurs in about 83% of patients with AIDS. Typically, the patient exhibits sadness, decreased self-esteem, hopelessness, withdrawal, and psychomotor retardation. Suicide rates are 66% higher among AIDS patients than among the general population — possibly because of associated brain lesions, a reaction to multiple losses, and feelings of social isolation, guilt, helplessness, and impending death.

The patient with AIDS may respond to his diagnosis with disbelief, numbness, and denial, followed by anger, emotional turmoil, suicidal ideation, and depressive symptoms. Such a patient faces a prolonged debility; an enormous need for physical, social, and financial assistance; and possibly family conflicts or conflicts about sexual identity. Depression may interfere with the patient's motivation to avoid infection and practice self-care measures.

*Cancer patients.* Depression occurs in about 45% of patients diagnosed with cancer. Probable causes include feelings of hopelessness and fear of pain and death.

*Demented patients.* Depression occurs in about 50% of patients with dementia. Of these, about 11% experience major depression. The patient's depression may stem from his awareness of his decreasing intellectual ability.

*Schizophrenic patients.* A patient with schizophrenia may show symptoms of major depression. Because he may lack the resources to seek emotional help, he runs a greater risk that depression will lead to suicide.

*Caregivers.* Depression affects as many as 81% of family members and other caregivers of patients with chronic cognitive or physical disorders. Among these caregivers, minor depression occurs twice as often as major depression. Members of lower socioeconomic and educational groups have fewer resources and are at greater risk of depression.

## Causes of depression
Mild, moderate, or severe depression can stem from various biological, psychological, and cognitive disorders. Other factors, including alcohol abuse and the use of certain drugs, can also precipitate depression.

*Biological causes.* Common biological factors that may increase a patient's risk of depression include genetic predisposition, hormonal fluctuations, biochemical changes, and organic disorders.

*Genetic predisposition.* Depression is as much as three times more prevalent in particular families than in the general population. And the family histories of prepubertal children with major depression include significantly more depression, psychosis, and alcoholism than those of children without depression.

Gender may also predispose a patient to certain types of depression. For instance, although manic-depressive illness tends to affect men and women equally, major depression is more than twice as prevalent in women.

*Hormonal fluctuations.* About 75% of new mothers experience some form of postpartum depression. For most, this takes the form of mild to moderate depression, known as the "baby blues." One out of 100 suffers severe postpartum psychosis, possibly caused by hormonal changes combined with physical stress, emotional conflict, and psychosocial stressors, such as an altered body image. Severe depression can lead to child abuse or suicide.

Premenstrual syndrome (PMS), also known as late luteal phase dysphoric disorder, is difficult to diagnose and assess. Yet 40% of menstruating women complain of dysphoric symptoms, and 10% of these women report that PMS affects their ability to function. Symptoms include irritability, depression, emotional lability, anxiety, and an increased potential for suicide.

*Biochemical changes.* In a patient who experiences depression, the brain handles neurotransmitters differently. For instance, in a patient with major depression, the neurotransmitters norepinephrine and dopamine are decreased. An excess of these neurotransmitters has been linked to mania. Currently, clinicians aren't certain what role acetylcholine and serotonin play in producing depression.

*Organic disorders.* Various organic disorders and chronic illnesses produce mild, moderate, or severe depression. These include metabolic and endocrine disorders, such as hypothyroidism, hyperthyroidism, and diabetes; infectious diseases, such as influenza, hepatitis, and encephalitis; degenerative diseases, such as Alzheimer's disease, multiple sclerosis, and multi-infarct dementia; and neoplastic diseases. Also, depression and mania may result from head trauma and regional cerebral blood flow.

**Psychological causes.** Depression may stem from a variety of psychological causes, including intrapsychic conflict, dependency, low self-esteem, feelings of powerlessness, unexpressed strong emotions, and guilt. Also, emotional trauma dating back to early childhood can contribute to depression among adults.

*Intrapsychic conflict.* This Freudian theory explains depression as "anger turned inward." That is, the anger a patient feels is directed not toward another person but toward himself. This anger is expressed as guilt and depression.

*Dependency.* Depression may result when a patient is overly dependent on another for feelings of self-worth. The depressed patient looks outward toward a more dominant person for validation of his existence, goals, and behavior.

*Low self-esteem.* A patient with a poor opinion of himself may easily become depressed by feelings of worthlessness, self-loathing, and inadequacy. A common cause of depression, low self-esteem can dangerously increase a patient's potential for suicide.

*Powerlessness.* A person may become depressed when he feels powerless to fulfill his wishes or control his life. For instance, an elderly patient's life is typically marked by personal loss — of income, loved ones, health, social contacts, and, above all, control. An overwhelming feeling of powerlessness may trigger a major depressive episode, which is the culmination of many years of mild, possibly unnoticed, depression.

*Unexpressed strong emotions.* A depressed patient may feel ambivalent or negative about certain aspects of his daily life. Instead of articulating these feelings, he turns them inward and expresses them as feelings of anger, worthlessness, guilt, and depression.

*Guilt.* A patient whose depression stems from guilt may have extremely high expectations for himself and an inability to fulfill them. Typically, he first experiences anxiety, then self-criticism, reduced self-esteem, and guilt. He also blames himself for a real or imagined loss and views himself as a failure who's hopeless and helpless.

*Early childhood losses and ineffectual bonding.* Emotional trauma in childhood and difficulties achieving autonomy and intimacy may cause depression in later years.

**Cognitive causes.** A depressed patient may experience dysfunctional thought processes that contribute to his depression. For instance, a patient who's a perfectionist may become depressed, unmotivated, and lethargic when his unrealistic standards of performance aren't met.

**Alcohol and other drugs.** Alcohol intoxication or withdrawal commonly produces depression. Also, various drugs cause depression as an adverse effect. Among the more common are barbiturates; antineoplastic agents, such as asparaginase; anticonvulsants, such as diazepam; and antiarrhythmics, such as disopyramide. Other drugs that may induce depression include centrally acting antihypertensives, such as reserpine (common in high dosages), methyldopa, and clonidine; beta-adrenergic blockers, such as propranolol; levodopa; indomethacin; cycloserine; corticosteroids; and oral contraceptives.

## Assessment

If you're caring for a patient who appears depressed or complains of depression, you'll need to perform a thorough assessment. Begin by taking a health history, focusing on the patient's psychosocial status and his

reaction to his illness and to hospitalization. As you assess the patient, observe his general appearance and behavior, and note any physical symptoms of depression he may have. Try to determine his suicide potential and, if necessary, take precautions to ensure his safety.

### Health history
Obtain or review the patient's health history to determine if his depression stems from his current illness, another medical condition, or any medications he's taking. Also explore drug and alcohol abuse. Review previous mental status evaluations, if any, and compare the findings with his current symptoms.

Then explore the patient's emotional status, self-image, environment, family history, and physical symptoms, using such communication skills as direct questioning, clarification, feedback, and expressions of support. If the patient is pregnant or has just given birth, try to determine her potential for postpartum depression.

**Emotional status.** Encourage the patient to discuss his feelings by asking broad, open-ended questions. Don't hurry the conversation: A depressed patient may think very slowly and need more time to respond. Use silence to help him collect his thoughts and work through his concerns.

Begin by asking the patient what's bothering him. How does he feel about his illness and hospitalization? How does his current mood differ from his usual mood? Can he pinpoint when the depression began? Has he ever had similar bouts of depression before? If so, does depression tend to strike at a particular time of the month or year? When he's feeling depressed, where does

## Assessing suicide risk

When you assess a patient's potential for suicide, consider these questions based on common risk factors.
• Is the patient a man or a woman? Although women make more suicide attempts, men are three times more likely to succeed.
• Is the patient younger than 19 or older than 45? Both teenagers and older patients are at higher risk.
• Is the patient single, separated, divorced, or widowed?
• Does the patient have an adequate support system?
• Is the patient an alcoholic?
• Is the patient depressed?
• Does the patient have a psychotic illness, especially one accompanied by delusions, hallucinations, and confusion?
• Does the patient have a serious or chronic illness?
• Has the patient tried to kill himself before?
• Does the patient have a simple, straightforward suicide plan that's likely to succeed?

he go and what does he do to feel better?

**Self-image.** Ask the patient to describe the way he feels about himself. What are his plans and dreams? Evaluate how realistic they are. Does he think his illness will interfere with those plans?

Is he generally satisfied with what he has accomplished in his work, relationships, and other interests? Ask about any changes in his social interactions, sleep patterns, ability to make decisions or concentrate, or normal activities.

**Environment.** Now ask the patient

about his environment. Has his life-style changed in the past month? Six months? Year? Find out how he feels about his role in the community and the resources available to him. Try to determine if he has an adequate support network to help him cope with his depression. If he has a long-term illness such as AIDS or cancer, find out if he knows about local support and self-help groups.

**Family history.** Find out about the patient's family — its patterns of interaction and characteristic responses to success and failure. What part does the patient feel he plays in his family life? Find out if other family members have been depressed. Also, determine whether anyone important to the patient has been sick or has died in the past year.

**Physical symptoms.** Because body functions slow down in response to depression, the patient may report constipation, diarrhea, anorexia, headache, dry mouth, hypotension, sleep disturbances, fatigue, lowered libido, and vague aches and pains. A suppressed immune system can predispose the patient to pneumonia, ulcers, urinary tract infections, viral infections, boils, pressure ulcers, and other infectious illnesses.

**Postpartum depression.** If your patient is pregnant or has just given birth, assess her potential for postpartum depression. Ask about her feelings toward the baby and the father. Does she have financial, interpersonal, or child care concerns?

If this isn't her first pregnancy, ask if she experienced postpartum depression before. If so, what were her symptoms? What type of treatment did she receive? What helped the most?

## General observations
A depressed patient may have a sullen expression and look older than his stated age. You also may note poor hygiene, an unkempt appearance, slouching, and a slow, shuffling gait. A depressed patient may have lost or gained a significant amount of weight over a short period of time.

*Behavior.* Typically, a depressed patient has little interest in his surroundings. He contributes little to conversations, has difficulty concentrating, and is preoccupied with himself and his negative feelings. Cognitive function, including short-term memory, is diminished.

A severely depressed patient may appear agitated, restless, and unable to sit still. His skin may be scratched or abraded from compulsive picking. He also may cry without tears, wring his hands, or laugh inappropriately.

The depressed patient may be sad and dejected or inappropriately elated (manic). Typically, a depressed patient is irritable, apathetic, and exhausted and lacks a sense of humor. He may express feelings of guilt or shame and low self-esteem. He also may assume responsibility for everything that goes wrong, exhibit hypochondriacal behavior, or say he feels as though he's a burden.

## Suicide potential
To determine your patient's suicide potential, ask him directly: "Have you ever thought of taking your own life? Do you feel like taking your life now?" Then find out if the patient has a simple, straightforward suicide plan that's likely to succeed. If so, what prevents him from acting on it? Does the patient receive any emotional support from family,

## Suicide: Separating fact from fiction

**Fiction:** Suicide typically strikes either the very rich or the very poor.

**Fact:** People from all socioeconomic groups kill themselves.

**Fiction:** Suicidal tendencies run in certain families.

**Fact:** Suicidal ideations and tendencies occur in individuals, not families.

**Fiction:** All suicidal people are mentally ill.

**Fact:** People who kill themselves are very unhappy—but not necessarily mentally ill.

**Fiction:** People who talk about committing suicide don't kill themselves.

**Fact:** About 80% of the people who commit suicide have given clear warnings of their intentions.

**Fiction:** You can't stop a person who's suicidal. He's intent on killing himself.

**Fact:** Most suicidal people can't decide whether they want to live or die. Timely intervention can save them.

**Fiction:** Once a patient starts to recover from severe depression, little risk of suicide remains.

**Fact:** Typically, people commit suicide during the first 3 months of their recovery from depression. As they improve, they gain the energy to carry out their suicidal intentions.

friends, or a therapist?

A patient with a low to moderate suicide potential is noticeably depressed but has some support system. He may have thoughts of suicide, but no specific plan. A patient with a high suicide potential feels profoundly hopeless and has little or no support system. He thinks about suicide frequently and has a plan that's likely to succeed. (See *Assessing suicide risk,* page 98.)

Keep in mind that not everyone who commits suicide is severely depressed. A patient may attempt suicide weeks or months after he begins to recover from severe depression. (See *Suicide: Separating fact from fiction,* page 99.)

---

# Intervention

If your patient appears depressed, you can intervene even if he doesn't have a medical diagnosis of depression. Make sure he receives enough nourishment and rest, and keep his environment free from stress and excessive stimulation. (See *Planning your care for a depressed patient.*)

Treatment for depression will vary with the type, characteristics, and severity. For instance, a patient who has seasonal affective disorder may improve after only a few days of phototherapy with bright artificial light. However, a patient with manic-depressive illness may require years of lithium therapy and counseling sessions.

Treating the underlying cause commonly helps a patient overcome depression that stems from a biological disorder. If the patient's depression doesn't have a treatable organic cause, therapeutic communi-

cation can help him identify what triggers his depressive moods and develop effective coping strategies.

If indicated, medication therapy, behavioral therapy, and cognitive therapy can also play important roles in overcoming depression. When other treatments fail, some patients may benefit from electroconvulsive therapy (ECT).

Finally, remember that your depressed patient may have suicidal tendencies and that as interventions start to improve his mood and make him feel more energetic, the risk of suicide increases. Assess him regularly and take appropriate steps to ensure his safety.

## Therapeutic communication

To establish therapeutic communication, you must show the patient that you care about his thoughts and behavior. So when you talk to him, sit down, show interest, touch his hand, and listen attentively. Accept his feelings as he expresses them, without imposing your own judgments or interpretations. For instance, if the patient says he feels lonely, you might respond by saying, "It seems difficult for you to deal with the loneliness." Avoid offering cliches, platitudes, or false reassurances. Also avoid appearing overly happy; this might make the patient feel that being unhappy is unacceptable.

Encourage the patient to express his thoughts and feelings by asking open-ended questions that require more than a one-word response. For instance, you might say something like "You look upset. Tell me what you're thinking about now." Accept his response with tolerance, respect, and concern, but don't allow him to repeat the same things over and over again. Instead, set a time limit for listening to him or have him write his feelings in a diary.

## Planning your care for a depressed patient

| NURSING DIAGNOSIS | EXPECTED OUTCOMES | INTERVENTIONS |
|---|---|---|
| Violence, potential for: Self-directed<br>• Feelings of guilt, inability to meet expectations, remorse over actions or thoughts, aggressive and hostile feelings, suicidal ideation, repressed hostility, anger turned inward | • Patient will remain safe during hospitalization.<br>• Patient will inform staff when he feels like harming himself. | • Place patient in a room near nurses' station.<br>• Remove all sharp objects from environment.<br>• Assess suicide potential every shift. Encourage patient to tell a staff member if he's feeling suicidal.<br>• Observe patient swallowing his medication.<br>• Assess need for continuous observation of patient on a one-to-one basis.<br>• Observe patient for signs of imminent suicide, such as giving away prized belongings or sudden behavioral changes (cheerfulness, relief, freedom from guilt).<br>• Closely observe patient for suicidal tendencies as antidepressant medication begins to take effect. |
| Self-esteem disturbance<br>• Feelings of worthlessness, excessive or inappropriate guilt, powerlessness, hopelessness; self-degradation<br>• In manic patients, grandiosity | • Patient will develop appropriate feelings of self-worth and express hopefulness. | • Encourage patient to take action, rather than waiting to feel better.<br>• Provide simple tasks or activities for patient to perform, and encourage his involvement in care.<br>• Gradually increase number and complexity of tasks or activities.<br>• Provide honest, positive feedback for each goal achieved.<br>• Encourage patient to solve problems independently. |
| Sleep pattern disturbance<br>• Insomnia, frequent brief naps, frequent night wakings, early waking (2 to 3 hours earlier than usual), difficulty falling asleep, hypersomnia<br>• In manic patients, decreased sleep requirements | • Patient will determine cause of sleep disturbance.<br>• Patient will sleep for increasing lengths of time or through the night.<br>• Patient will be awake to participate in daily activities. | • Assess patient's sleep pattern, and note time and circumstances of disturbance.<br>• Discuss possible causes of sleep disturbance.<br>• Teach relaxation techniques.<br>• Encourage patient to avoid caffeine and foods that produce stimulant effect before going to sleep.<br>• Provide a nonstimulating environment during the evening to promote sleep.<br>• Give medications as needed, and note their effectiveness.<br>*(continued)* |

## Planning your care for a depressed patient *(continued)*

| NURSING DIAGNOSIS | EXPECTED OUTCOMES | INTERVENTIONS |
|---|---|---|
| Social isolation<br>• Isolation, reclusiveness, decreased libido, unwillingness to start conversation, monosyllabic speech<br>• In manic patients, nervousness, hypersexuality, loud talking | • Patient will identify sources of impaired social interaction.<br>• Patient will engage in socially acceptable behaviors.<br>• Patient will interact effectively with others. | • Initiate therapeutic nurse-patient relationship.<br>• Assess source of impaired social interaction, and discuss ways to alter behavior.<br>• Teach methods that lead to socially acceptable interactions.<br>• Provide a safe, structured environment. |
| Self-care deficit<br>• Disheveled appearance, poor hygiene and grooming, body odor, unwillingness to change clothes or get dressed, unwillingness to take a bath or wash<br>• In manic patients, preference for bright colors, excessive jewelry or make-up, provocative clothing | • Patient will demonstrate improvement in self-care. | • Assess patient's ability to perform activities of daily living (ADLs) independently.<br>• Encourage patient to participate in ADLs.<br>• Set small goals initially.<br>• Provide positive reinforcement for participation in self-care.<br>• Support and reinforce patient's efforts toward independence.<br>• Discourage use of inappropriate, bizarre dress and make-up by setting consistent, non-punitive limits. |
| Altered nutrition<br>• Poor appetite, lack of interest in eating or compulsive eating—especially of high-carbohydrate foods | • Patient will have a balanced diet.<br>• Patient's weight will begin to approach normal limits for his body structure.<br>• Patient will recognize importance of proper nutrition.<br>• Patient will focus on emotional source of dysfunctional eating.<br>• Patient will begin to recover physically from eating disturbance. | • Monitor food and fluid intake.<br>• Weigh patient in morning before breakfast without shoes, as ordered.<br>• Teach patient importance of adequate nutritional intake.<br>• Provide supportive counseling to address issues associated with altered nutrition.<br>• Support dietitian's interventions. |

***Pinpoint what triggers depression.*** Help the patient identify stressors that trigger mild, moderate, or severe depression. Sometimes, a seemingly minor event can trigger a major depressive reaction, perhaps by reminding the patient of past emotional trauma. Understanding the reason for his reaction may help him resolve the issues that are causing his depression.

***Help the patient cope.*** Determine how the patient deals with depression and, if necessary, teach him more effective ways to cope. If his condition permits, encourage him to follow an exercise program instead of sitting around and brooding. Exercise increases neurotransmitter turnover, produces a sense of mastery over a task, and often yields positive reinforcement from others. For some patients, it can be as effective as antidepressant therapy.

Encourage the patient to assert his opinions and make decisions. This will help promote feelings of control and self-worth. Also, encourage him to acknowledge the anger that underlies his depression and help him express it safely. For instance, plan activities that provide a controlled outlet for anger. To help him overcome feelings of helplessness, plan activities that he can succeed at and teach him to solve problems constructively. Help foster feelings of competence by focusing on past and present experiences in which he was successful.

Encourage the patient to socialize and participate in simple activities to increase his self-esteem. If appropriate, suggest volunteer work, or refer the patient for family therapy or group therapy. Becoming involved with other people may help the patient counteract loneliness, which often underlies depression.

If the patient refuses to do anything to help himself, try to understand and respect his feelings, but encourage him to participate in physical or social activities. As you gain the patient's trust, he'll be more willing to go along with your suggestions.

## Drug therapy
Depending on the type of depression, a doctor may order drug therapy. In such cases, you'll administer the prescribed drug and assess its effects. Also, you must make sure the patient understands when to take his medication and which adverse effects to look for.

*Antidepressants.* For a patient suf-

fering a major depressive episode, the treatment of choice is antidepressant drug therapy. The most commonly used antidepressants, tricyclic antidepressants enhance norepinephrine's release by blocking its reabsorption. Tetracyclic antidepressants work in a similar manner.

Other commonly used antidepressants include fluoxetine (Prozac), which blocks the uptake of serotonin, and bupropion (Wellbutrin), which prevents the uptake of norepinephrine and dopamine.

A doctor will prescribe a monoamine oxidase (MAO) inhibitor only as a last resort because of the severe adverse effects these drugs can cause. They combat depression by blocking the action of an enzyme that breaks down norepinephrine and the related neurotransmitter serotonin. Thus, these highly toxic drugs increase the amount of norepinephrine in the synapse.

If the doctor does prescribe an MAO inhibitor, teach the patient to avoid foods that contain tyramine, such as wine and cheese, and to check with his doctor before taking any other drug. MAO inhibitors can interact with tyramine and sympathomimetics to cause hypertensive crisis. (See *Common antidepressant medications,* pages 104 and 105.)

*Lithium.* For a patient with manic-depressive illness or cyclothymia, a doctor may order lithium. Although the exact mechanism of action isn't clear, lithium apparently alters certain neurotransmitters and sodium exchange in the brain.

When initiating lithium therapy, obtain weekly blood levels of the medication until it reaches a therapeutic level (1 to 1.5 mEq/liter). Then obtain monthly blood lithium levels until therapy ends. Take

*(Text continues on page 106.)*

# Common antidepressant medications

## Tricyclic antidepressants

amitriptyline hydrochloride (Elavil)

**Average adult daily dosage**
75 to 300 mg

**Adverse reactions**
Arrhythmias, dizziness, dry mouth, headache, mydriasis, postural hypotension, reflex tachycardia, seizures, tinnitus

imipramine hydrochloride (Tofranil)

**Average adult daily dosage**
75 to 300 mg

**Adverse reactions**
Arrhythmias, dry mouth, hypersensitivity, myocardial infarction, seizures, tremor, urine retention

amoxapine (Asendin)

**Average adult daily dosage**
50 to 300 mg

**Adverse reactions**
Arrhythmias, blurred vision, dizziness, dry mouth, nervousness, peripheral neuropathy, postural hypotension, sedation, seizures, weakness

nortriptyline hydrochloride (Pamelor)

**Average adult daily dosage**
50 to 100 mg

**Adverse reactions**
Dizziness, drowsiness, ECG changes, heart block, paralytic ileus, photosensitivity, postural hypotension, reflex tachycardia, sweating

desipramine hydrochloride (Norpramin)

**Average adult daily dosage**
50 to 300 mg

**Adverse reactions**
Arrhythmias, dry mouth, ECG changes, extrapyramidal symptoms, increased intraocular pressure, seizures

protriptyline hydrochloride (Vivactil)

**Average adult daily dosage**
15 to 60 mg

**Adverse reactions**
Arrhythmias, blurred vision, constipation, memory impairment, seizures, sinus tachycardia, urine retention

doxepin hydrochloride (Sinequan)

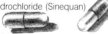

**Average adult daily dosage**
75 to 150 mg

**Adverse reactions**
Anorexia, arrhythmias, constipation, dry mouth, excitation, hypotension, palpitations, seizures

trimipramine maleate (Surmontil)

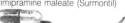

**Average adult daily dosage**
75 to 200 mg

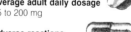

**Adverse reactions**
Congestive heart failure, dry mouth, extrapyramidal symptoms, hypersensitivity, mydriasis, tachycardia

### Tetracyclic antidepressant

maprotiline hydrochloride (Ludiomil)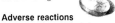
**Average adult daily dosage**
50 to 225 mg

**Adverse reactions**
Excitation, heart block, hypersensitivity, mydriasis, palpitations, seizures (high incidence)

### Monoamine oxidase (MAO) inhibitors

isocarboxazid (Marplan)

**Average adult daily dosage**
10 to 50 mg

**Adverse reactions**
Abdominal pain, arrhythmias, discolored urine, dry mouth, hyperreflexia, hypotension, muscle twitching, paradoxical hypertension

phenelzine sulfate (Nardil)

**Average adult daily dosage**
15 to 75 mg

**Adverse reactions**
Fatigue, hypotension, mania, memory impairment, nervousness, orthostatic hypotension, weight changes

tranylcypromine sulfate (Parnate)

**Average adult daily dosage**
10 to 60 mg

**Adverse reactions**
Arrhythmias, dizziness, dry mouth, hypotension, jaundice, peripheral edema, vertigo

### Other antidepressants

bupropion (Wellbutrin)

**Average adult daily dosage**
225 to 450 mg

**Adverse reactions**
Seizures

fluoxetine (Prozac)

**Average adult daily dosage**
40 to 80 mg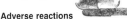

**Adverse reactions**
Anorexia, diarrhea, dry mouth, headache, insomnia, nausea, nervousness, weight loss

trazodone hydrochloride (Desyrel)

**Average adult daily dosage**
50 to 600 mg

**Adverse reactions**
Diarrhea, drowsiness, dry mouth, hypotension, insomnia, light-headedness, priapism

blood samples 8 to 12 hours after the last dose.

The usual lithium dosage is 600 to 1,800 mg daily. During therapy, make sure that the patient isn't on a low-sodium diet and that he maintains an adequate but not excessive fluid intake because sodium and fluid levels affect lithium levels. Also, monitor him for signs of toxicity, including nausea, vomiting, abdominal cramps, thirst, polyuria, and impaired coordination. Notify the doctor immediately if these signs develop.

### Behavioral therapy

This form of therapy involves assessing the patient's behavior and altering patterns that lead to depression. Depending on the nature of the patient's depression, he may benefit from individual, group, family, or environmental therapy.

*Individual therapy.* By using positive reinforcement, individual therapy helps change the depressed patient's behavior patterns. This therapy involves asking the patient to help plan his treatment and to set realistic goals.

If the patient can't participate in planning, develop a treatment plan for him and explain what you expect him to do. Encourage him to accomplish small tasks that he can complete without difficulty. For example, if he feels too depressed to eat a whole meal, encourage him to try eating just a few bites. Provide positive reinforcement for any improvement he shows. This therapy combats helplessness and gives the patient a feeling of control, thus improving self-esteem.

*Group therapy.* In many cases, a patient's problems and coping methods are more apparent to his peers than to himself. Sharing anger, frustration, and concerns with others who are experiencing similar problems builds feelings of trust and counteracts isolation. Hearing how others overcame their problems may foster optimism.

An assertiveness training or communication group may help a depressed patient learn how to express his wants, needs, and desires — instead of getting angry and turning the anger inward. Peer self-help groups are especially effective for those with cancer, cardiac disease, and AIDS, providing both guidance and an opportunity for patients to help each other, thus improving self-esteem.

*Family therapy.* If family tensions cause or aggravate the patient's depression, family therapy may help resolve the conflict. Such therapy can also teach family members effective coping methods, enabling them to help the patient overcome his depression — and to avoid becoming depressed themselves.

*Environmental therapy.* With this type of therapy, the patient has opportunities and resources for *physical diversions,* such as exercise sessions, volley ball, or bowling; *mental diversions,* such as card games, board games, pool, or television; and *contemplative diversions,* such as meditating, journal writing, or correspondence. To be effective, environmental therapy requires a consistent routine and understanding staff members who have enough self-awareness to care for the patient objectively.

### Cognitive therapy

This form of therapy uses special techniques to alter thought patterns that commonly cause or exacerbate depression. For instance, the thought-stopping technique sets limits on destructive thinking, thereby counteracting feelings of hopelessness. For some patients, the results can be even more effective than antidepressant medication.

To use thought stopping, first help the patient increase his awareness of when he's having negative thoughts. Then tell him to stop thinking the thought and examine it logically. Help him find alternative problem-solving techniques. For instance, if he finds himself dwelling on a mistake he made, have him switch from focusing on what he did wrong to what positive steps he can take if the situation arises again. Encourage him to think positive thoughts—for instance, have him focus on his accomplishments. This not only builds self-esteem but also gives the patient an opportunity to see the situation from another perspective.

### Electroconvulsive therapy

This controversial treatment uses an electric current to induce seizures. Although the mechanism of action is unclear, ECT is known to help certain depressed patients—especially those who've tried various antidepressants unsuccessfully and elderly patients who can't tolerate antidepressants. Most patients require 8 to 12 treatments; some may need monthly treatments to prevent depression from recurring.

To prepare a patient for ECT, instruct him to restrict food and fluids after midnight on the day of treatment. Reinforce the doctor's explanation of the procedure and answer the patient's questions. Also, advise him of the possible adverse effects, including confusion, headache, and short-term memory loss. Monitor vital signs during and after treatment.

### Suicide prevention

When caring for a depressed patient, always consider the risk of suicide and regularly assess him for suicidal tendencies. If appropriate, encourage the patient to sign a contract stating that he'll contact a staff member immediately if he feels suicidal.

Place the patient in a room near the nurses' station, and know where he is and what he's doing at all times. With some patients, this will require one-to-one monitoring. Always have someone accompany a suicidal patient off the unit.

Ensure the patient's safety by removing objects he could use to harm himself, such as razors, belts, and electrical cords. Also, make sure he swallows prescribed medications you give him. Otherwise, he may try to hoard them for use in a suicide attempt.

Keep in mind that in-hospital suicide attempts typically occur when the staff-to-patient ratio is low—for instance, between shifts, during evening and night shifts, or when a critical event, such as a code, draws attention away from the patient. Also remember that the risk of suicide is greatest when depression lifts and the patient starts to feel more energetic.

# Evaluation

Effective interventions will help the patient reach several goals. He'll be able to talk about his depression and describe the signs and symptoms he's experiencing. He'll also be able to recognize emotional and behavioral changes that signal the approach of a depressive episode. Such changes include a failure to so-

## When to consult a mental health professional

According to the *Diagnostic and Statistical Manual of Mental Disorders,* 3rd edition (revised), you should consult a mental health professional if your patient is suicidal or if he exhibits five or more of these symptoms for 2 weeks or more:
• depressed mood most of the time
• apathy
• significant weight loss or gain resulting from a change in appetite
• insomnia or hypersomnia
• psychomotor agitation or retardation
• fatigue or loss of energy
• low self-esteem, feelings of worthlessness, or excessive or inappropriate guilt
• diminished ability to think
• feelings of hopelessness or helplessness
• recurrent thoughts of death
• suicidal ideations or plan.

cialize, to exercise as usual, and to regularly attend support group meetings.

Moreover, the patient will be able to identify what triggers his depression, what alleviates it, and what emotional resources and supports are available to him. He'll also know when he can control depression himself and when he needs help.

As his depression decreases, the patient will perform more personal hygiene functions, appear neater and cleaner, sleep better, and feel more energetic. He'll also begin to eat more nutritious meals, stabilize his weight within the ideal range, enjoy more activities, and exercise regularly. As well, the patient will begin to initiate conversations, socialize and smile more, hold his head erect, walk with a quicker step, have fewer physical complaints, and project a more optimistic view of life.

### Suicide precautions
Did your precautions and therapeutic interventions keep the suicidal patient safe? Have his suicidal tendencies ceased?

If, despite precautions, a patient on your unit attempts suicide, discuss the incident with other staff members. Share concerns and explore whether additional therapeutic interventions are needed.

### Requesting a consultation
Depending on the circumstances, you may request a consultation at any point in the nursing process. Typically, you'll assess, intervene, and evaluate the patient before consulting with a psychiatrist or psychiatric clinical nurse specialist.

Sometimes, though, you'll request a consultation earlier—for instance, if the patient has, or may have, a psychiatric diagnosis. Also, if your patient becomes suicidal, have him evaluated immediately by a psychiatric clinical nurse specialist or a psychiatrist. Notify the patient's doctor of this change. (See *When to consult a mental health professional.*)

If the patient continues to show signs and symptoms of depression or mania for 2 or more weeks, or if he just isn't responding to interventions, you should also seek a consultation. Request help as well if you or other members of the health care team feel frustrated or hopeless when working with a patient. If you or your co-workers feel this way, chances are the patient does, too. A psychiatric clinical nurse specialist or a psychiatrist can assess the patient and work with the health care team to formulate diagnoses and interventions.

## Suggested readings

Beck, A.T., et al. "Relationship Between Hopelessness and Ultimate Suicide: A Replication with Psychiatric Outpatients," *American Journal of Psychiatry* 147(2):190-95, February 1990.

Beck, C.K., et al. *Mental Health-Psychiatric Nursing: A Holistic Life-Cycle Approach,* 2nd ed. St. Louis: C.V. Mosby Co., 1988.

Busch, P., and Perrin, K. "Post-partum Depression: Assessing Risk, Restoring Balance," *RN* 52(8):46-49, August 1989.

Denmark, F., and Kabatznick, R. "Women and Suicide," in *Affective Disorders.* Edited by Flach, F. New York: W.W. Norton & Co., 1988.

*Diagnostic and Statistical Manual of Mental Disorders,* 3rd ed., revised. Washington, D.C.: American Psychiatric Association, 1987.

Dura, J., et al. "Chronic Stress and Depressive Disorders in Older Adults," *Journal of Abnormal Psychology* 99(3):284-90, August 1990.

Glod, C. "Seasonal Affective Disorder: A New Light?" *Journal of Psychosocial Nursing and Mental Health Services* 29(3):38-39, March 1991.

Hall, J., and Stevens, P. "AIDS: A Guide to Suicide Assessment," *Archives of Psychiatric Nursing* 2(2):115-20, April 1988.

Keane, S., and Sells, S. "Recognizing Depression in the Elderly," *Journal of Gerontological Nursing* 16(1):21-25, January 1989.

Keitner, G., and Miller, I. "Family Functioning and Major Depression: An Overview," *American Journal of Psychiatry* 147(9):1128-37, September 1990.

McEnany, G. "Nursing the Mind: Managing Mood Disorders," *RN* 53(9):28-33, September 1990.

McEnany, G. "Psychobiological Indices of Bipolar Mood Disorder: Future Trends in Nursing Care," *Archives of Psychiatric Nursing* 4(1):29-38, February 1990.

Perko, J., and Kreigh, H. *Psychiatric and Mental Health Nursing,* 3rd ed. Norwalk, Conn.: Appleton & Lange, 1988.

Schmidt, P., et al. "State-Dependent Alterations in the Perception of Life Events in Menstrual-Related Mood Disorders," *American Journal of Psychiatry* 147(2):230-34, February 1990.

Simmons-Alling, S. "Genetic Implications for Major Affective Disorders," *Archives of Psychiatric Nursing* 4(1):67-71, February 1990.

Siomopoulos, V. "When Patients Commit Suicide, Risk Factors to Watch For," *Postgraduate Medicine* 88(3):205-13, September 1, 1990.

Wilson, H.S., and Kneisl, C.R. *Psychiatric Nursing,* 3rd ed. Menlo Park, Calif.: Addison-Wesley Publishing Co., 1988.

# 7
# GRIEF

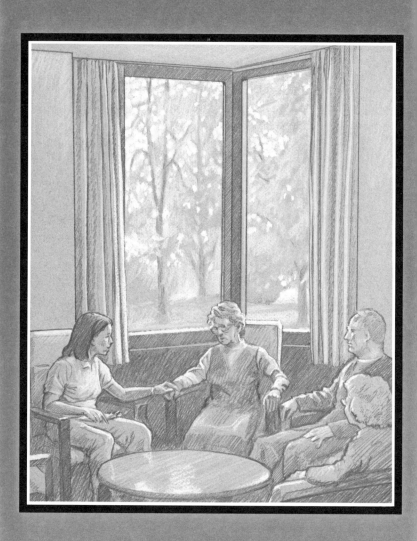

"What do I say to a dying patient?" "What if I say the wrong thing and upset him?" "How do I comfort a grieving family?" "Should I show my emotions at bedside?" "How should I manage my own feelings about death?"

These and many other questions arise when you care for patients and families facing death or another significant loss. At times, you may feel conflicting emotions. You want to comfort the patient and his family, but you aren't always sure how to do it.

This chapter will help give you the confidence you need to care for a dying patient and his family. It reviews the grieving process, compares adaptive and maladaptive grief responses, and explores the complexities of unresolved grief. The chapter also discusses how to assess a grieving patient and how to intervene effectively. Of course, before you can help others cope with a loss, you must come to terms with your own feelings about death and dying, loss and grieving. This chapter helps you put those feelings into perspective so that you can provide your patient with understanding care.

# Understanding grief

Grieving allows a person to gradually accept changes that are beyond his control. Anyone who experiences a significant loss will need to grieve before he can move on to reorganize and reestablish his life. Such a loss may be the death of a loved one, of course. But it may also be the loss of health, stamina, and autonomy associated with aging or the loss of

a body part or of normal function brought on by injury, surgery, or disease. (See *Patients who grieve*, page 112.)

Grieving may begin when a patient first anticipates a potential loss or after the loss occurs. Grieving response patterns will vary greatly, depending on a person's cultural background, religious beliefs, and personality as well as the extent of the loss.

## Types of grief

Anticipatory grief occurs before a loss that a person perceives as inevitable. Unlike grief that occurs during or after a loss and diminishes with time, anticipatory grief may increase in intensity as the expected loss draws near. Sometimes — particularly when the loss is delayed — a person can completely expend his anticipatory grief, leading to emotional detachment and fewer signs of acute grief when the actual loss occurs.

The nature of the loss also determines the type of grief a person experiences. For example, a person may view the death of an elderly or long-suffering loved one as a blessing but may experience acute grief following the unexpected death of a young child. When a sudden death or another unexpected loss occurs, those involved must handle the situation without any preparation or warning. This can create an immobilizing sense of unreality about the loss.

## Grieving responses

People who must deal with a significant loss experience similar emotional reactions. By understanding these characteristic reactions you'll be better able to assess and help a patient and his family as they try to adapt to their loss.

## Patients who grieve

Anyone who experiences a significant loss will need to grieve. This includes patients in the following situations:
☐ A patient receives a serious medical diagnosis and must adjust to its impact on himself and his family.
☐ A patient loses a body part or experiences a change in normal physical function and, together with his family, must learn to accept a changed body image.
☐ A chronicallly ill patient and his family must adjust to the exacerbations and remissions of chronic illness.
☐ A dying patient and his family must learn to accept his impending death.

**Anticipatory response.** The best-known theory on the grieving process was established by Elisabeth Kübler-Ross. She described five emotional responses, all related to the grieving process: denial, anger, bargaining, depression, and acceptance. Although these are the stages a dying person experiences, they also apply to any person who's facing a significant loss.

Remember that most patients don't progress in an orderly manner from one phase of the grieving process to the next. For example, a dying patient experiencing anger about his impending death may project it onto someone or something else while denying that he's terminally ill. (See *Recognizing the five stages of grief.*)

*Denial.* Initially, a patient may respond to his impending death or loss with overwhelming shock and disbelief. He rejects the reality of the situation as a temporary defense against this catastrophic loss. He

might say or think something like "That's impossible; this can't be happening to me." He may even have physical responses, such as sweating, pallor, faintness, nausea, and confusion.

*Anger.* Feelings of rage, envy, resentment, and bitterness naturally occur when a terminal illness or major loss disrupts a patient's life. The patient may wonder "Why me?" He also may display impatience, uncooperativeness, and helplessness — all of which can impede nursing assessment and care.

*Bargaining.* In this final attempt to avoid the reality of the impending death or loss, the patient tries to strike a bargain with God or another higher power for health or extended life. Typically, the patient is depressed and exhausted. The bargaining stage usually doesn't affect the patient's behavior during assessment and interventions.

*Depression.* In this stage, the patient experiences grief for the impending death or loss. He may be quiet, withdrawn, and melancholy as he gradually accepts reality.

*Acceptance.* A patient who has learned to accept the reality of his impending death or loss displays emotional readiness for the inevitable loss. He may seem contemplative, serene, and willing to talk about his condition.

**Survivor's response.** After the death or loss has occurred, the survivor will typically experience three grieving phases — disequilibrium, disorganization, and reorganization.

*Disequilibrium.* Initially, the survivor may not comprehend — or even

## Recognizing the five stages of grief

The grieving process consists of five stages—denial, anger, bargaining, depression, and acceptance. Keep in mind that your patient may not experience these stages in sequence.

| STAGE | SIGNS AND SYMPTOMS |
|---|---|
| Denial | • Overwhelming shock and disbelief<br>• Rejection of reality<br>• Sweating, pallor, faintness, nausea, confusion |
| Anger | • Impatience<br>• Uncooperativeness<br>• Bitterness<br>• Helplessness<br>• Sarcasm<br>• Increasing awareness |
| Bargaining | • Depression and exhaustion<br>• Final attempt to avoid reality<br>• Periodic physical symptoms, such as shortness of breath and weakness |
| Depression | • Withdrawal<br>• Melancholy<br>• Gradual acceptance of reality |
| Acceptance | • Contemplativeness and serenity<br>• Ability to talk about loss |

acknowledge—the reality of the loss. He may display shock, bewilderment, numbness, disbelief, and denial. He also may cry, sigh, or scream in protest—an important step toward recognizing that the loss has occurred.

Physical expressions of disequilibrium may include a loss of appetite, fatigue, empty feelings, tightness in the throat, shortness of breath, poor memory, difficulty concentrating, and sleep disturbances. The survivor may be preoccupied with anger, guilt, or fantasies of the deceased. He may express anger toward himself, the deceased, family members, or health care professionals whom he associates with the death. He also may direct his anger toward God or another higher power for allowing the death to occur.

*Disorganization.* This stage is characterized by the realization that the loss is permanent. It generally occurs a few weeks after the loss and can continue for several months. Typically, the survivor feels lonely, afraid, and helpless. He limits social interaction and may have difficulty performing daily activities. Persistent thoughts of the deceased may increase at night, causing sleep disturbances and a heightened sense of isolation. Physical symptoms of stress associated with disequilibrium may persist.

*Reorganization.* When the survivor

## Comparing adaptive and maladaptive grief responses

A positive, or adaptive, grief response involves acknowledging and mourning the loss, and gradually becoming detached enough to move on with life. A negative, or maladaptive, response stems from the patient's failure to resolve his grief and leads to prolonged depression or mania.

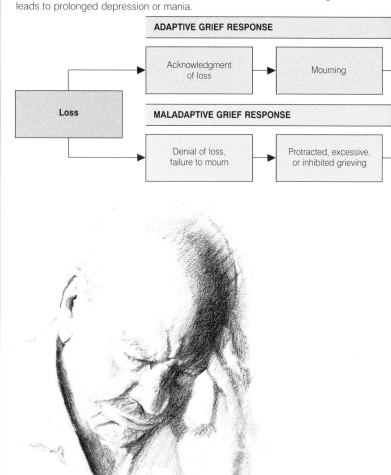

reaches this stage, he can accept the loss and form new goals and relationships. The survivor may incorporate the values and behaviors of the deceased in a satisfying way and enjoy life. This phase may begin from 6 months to 2 years after the loss.

### Unresolved grief
When a person can't acknowledge a significant loss or experience its

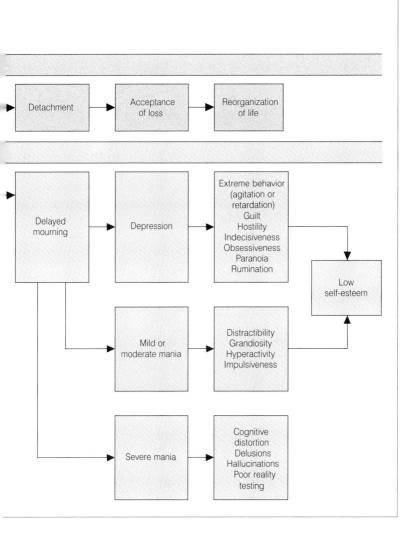

sadness, his grief is unresolved. The intensity of the loss may be so overwhelming that the person resorts to maladaptive or self-destructive behaviors. For instance, he may try to avoid facing the loss by increasing his activities, abusing alcohol or drugs, overeating, or acting impulsively. Prolonged reactions of anger and aggression toward himself and others may occur.

The most common reaction to unresolved grief is mild, chronic depression that commonly goes unnoticed. The person may withdraw from friends, stop going to church, feel guilty in various situations, and suffer various aches and pains. (See *Comparing adaptive and maladaptive grief responses,* pages 114 and 115.)

***Causes of unresolved grief.*** People fail to grieve for many reasons. The "strong one" in a family may offer support to everyone else but miss the opportunity to deal with his own grief. Guilt arising from feelings of ambivalence about the deceased person's death may also delay grief. As well, mourning may be more difficult when the survivor perceives the deceased person as an extension of himself; he may feel he has lost a part of himself and will never be the same again.

The loss of more than one person can produce overwhelming shock and may also impede grieving. Or a person may resist mourning because of a fear of being looked upon as weak, a concern about hurting other people, a fear of losing control, or a feeling of guilt over the satisfying release of crying.

# Assessment

You'll use the same basic techniques when you assess all grieving patients. However, you'll need to modify your assessment somewhat, depending on whether your patient is grieving for himself or for a loved one. You'll also need to tailor the assessment to your patient's grieving response and to the particular phase he's experiencing.

A patient who's denying his own or a family member's condition presents a paradoxical situation: You need to discuss the reality of the situation with him, yet he won't acknowledge it. In such a case, keep in mind that denial helps a person maintain his emotional equilibrium. Don't try to force him to admit the situation exists, but don't hold out false hope for recovery either. Instead, gently proceed with the assessment at a pace your patient can tolerate.

## Dying patient
Assess a dying patient to identify his problems and his physical, emotional, and spiritual needs. Working with the patient, establish realistic and measurable treatment goals.

***Physical needs.*** Assess the patient's physical condition to determine his response to the terminal illness. Determine his ability to perform activities of daily living. Also note his mobility, sleep patterns, and nutritional, fluid, and elimination status. Is he having problems coping with the physical limitations of the disease? Keep in mind that resolving the patient's physical concerns will allow him more energy to deal with the emotional ones.

Determine whether the patient is in pain. Remember, pain can cause fear, anxiety, and a feeling of helplessness — which, in turn, can bring on more pain.

***Emotional needs.*** Try to determine how the patient feels about his impending death. His attitude will have been shaped partly by his own health and personal history and partly by his reactions to the deaths of family members and friends. Listen carefully for any direct or indirect references to his death. Integrate the topic into the conversation when you think he's ready to talk about it.

What effect does he think his illness and death will have on his family? What are his greatest concerns about helping his family cope? Does he have problems he'd like to resolve before he dies? Does he feel his family will provide adequate support to help him through the dying process?

The attitudes of your patient's friends and family members toward death will affect how much help they can give him. Observe how the patient interacts with family members. Talk with them, and describe in your notes their potential for helping the patient accept his condition.

Explore the patient's final wishes. Determine what he'd like to do before he dies, how he'd like to die, and who he wants to be with him when he dies.

*Spiritual needs.* Determine how the patient's religious beliefs influence his grieving response. Spiritual strength may help the patient cope with the stress of loss. Find out which religious resources or rituals he feels will help him cope.

### Patient losing a body part
Determine the patient's body image — his perception of his body and its physical capabilities. Body image contributes to a person's overall sense of identity and affects both the way he treats his body and his anxiety level when dealing with others. Severe anxiety can result from a failure to adjust one's body image when a natural development, a disease, or an injury changes the body.

How does the patient feel the lost body part will affect his perception of himself? What's his greatest concern about the loss? How does he

think that family members and others will respond? Is he afraid that people will have a lower opinion of his worth? Does he fear that his spouse will leave him because of his new limitations? Find out whether the patient is receiving adequate support from family members and spiritual resources.

### Family members
If possible, try to determine the nature of the patient's family relationships before the death or other loss occurs. Do family interactions seem nurturing and caring, or tense and argumentative? Do family members appear to accept the patient's condition, or are they reluctant to discuss it? Do they have any unresolved problems with the patient?

After the death or other loss occurs, assess the family's coping skills. How do their religious beliefs influence their ability to grieve? Do they have adequate support to deal with the crisis?

Determine how the family members are expressing their grief. Grieving is commonly accompanied by depression, which may appear as changes in behavior (apathy, self-deprecation, anger, inertia), changes in thought processes (confusion, disorientation, poor judgment), or somatic complaints (appetite loss, constipation, insomnia).

### Patient with previously unresolved grief
If your patient has experienced a significant loss within the past 2 years — the death of a loved one, for instance — begin your assessment by trying to determine if he has resolved his grief. Find out, for instance, if he refused to attend religious or funeral services for the loved one. Observe the patient's behavior as you interview him. Does

his voice quaver or do tears come to his eyes when he talks about his loved one? Does he dwell on themes of loss?

Determine whether the patient has chronic grief symptoms, such as persistent guilt, depression, and lowered self-esteem. If so, do his symptoms worsen on the anniversary of the death or during holidays? Do relatively minor events trigger symptoms of grief? A failure to resolve an earlier grief experience can exacerbate the current crisis, causing a pathologic grief reaction.

Carefully assess the patient's suicide potential. Has he considered suicide as a method of joining his loved one? Does he receive support from family, friends, or a therapist? Have his relationships with his family and friends changed since the loss?

# Intervention

Before you can help a grieving patient, you need to examine your own feelings about death and dying, grieving and loss. Then, depending on the patient's specific needs, you may use therapeutic communication, help to relieve his pain, or help to build an adequate support network.

## Examining your feelings
Your personal attitudes and beliefs about grieving and loss influence your relationship with your patient. For example, if you've recently lost a loved one and haven't effectively grieved for him, listening to a patient's expressions of grief may revive your own emotional pain and interfere with your ability to give nursing care.

Sometimes, you may fear showing sympathy and emotion at the bedside because you don't want to appear out of control. But remember, crying is a controlled way of showing and releasing emotion. Uncontrolled sobbing, however, may upset the patient and won't be therapeutically effective.

You may also feel helpless when caring for a dying patient. If so, remind yourself that you can help best by providing comfort and projecting a caring, therapeutic attitude.

## Therapeutic communication
To help the patient and his family grieve effectively, build on the therapeutic relationship you established during your assessment. With words and gestures, let the patient and his family know that their feelings, thoughts, and needs are important to you.

Don't offer false comfort or make light of the patient's condition. Provide honest information and explanations while maintaining an atmosphere of security and caring. Avoid statements that minimize the emotional pain the patient and his family are experiencing. For instance, don't say, "It could be worse" or "Don't be sad; life will go on." Simply acknowledging their loss and listening to them can be more therapeutic than giving advice.

Many people are frightened by the grieving process and want to know if it's normal. If needed, provide the patient and his family with information about the stages of grieving and the length of time the process usually takes.

*Communicating with the patient.* At the beginning of the crisis, allow the patient to grieve without unnecessary interference. Help him to express fears and anxieties at his own pace, rather than forcing the issue. Accept his expressions of anger and guilt without being defensive or judgmental.

Initially, when the patient doesn't want to talk, just sit quietly with him for a short time. Don't rush him or attempt to figure out what he's going to say before he says it. Sometimes accepting a few moments of silence until you or the patient feels like talking again can be therapeutic. Touch or hug the patient if it seems appropriate, but be alert for clues that he finds this uncomfortable.

When possible, allow the patient to make decisions that affect his life or the dying process.

*Encouraging communication.* If, after a time, a patient continues refusing to communicate with you or a colleague, he may need more help to confront the feelings and thoughts he's trying to avoid. Encourage him to discuss the loss. For example, say something like "It must have been difficult for you when you heard about your diagnosis." Reassure him that he will not cry indefinitely, lose control permanently, or go crazy. Explain that grieving is a normal, necessary process.

**Communicating with the family.** Allow family members to express their feelings before and after the loss occurs. Don't overlook their need to grieve because of your focus on the patient.

Encourage communication between the patient and his family. Provide information about the treatment plan, and allow family members to assist with care when possible. Involving them in the care of the dying person will decrease their anxiety and promote the patient's comfort.

Sometimes a family member may express anger at the loved one for dying or for causing emotional pain. This can occur even when the relationship between them is loving and caring. Such expressions of anger may also be directed at you or another staff member. If this occurs, try to be understanding.

After the patient dies, share last-minute details about his death with the family, as appropriate. For example, you might say that the patient was quiet and comfortable right before he died, if that's what you observed. Ask if family members want to spend time alone with their loved one. Do they want a member of the clergy present? Do they want an undertaker to be notified? When possible, offer the family a private environment outside of the patient's room to help them express their grief. (See *Helping the bereaved family cope,* page 120.)

### Pain relief
Using analgesics and comfort measures, relieve the patient's pain based on his wishes. Some patients want to be completely pain-free, whereas others can tolerate a minimal amount of discomfort. Ideally, the patient should be as comfortable as he wants to be while remaining alert and in control.

### Support network
A grieving patient and his family may need emotional and financial support. Help them develop a support network by referring them to appropriate community groups or organizations, such as local units of the American Cancer Society or American Heart Association, or a community mental health center. The hospital social services department can also help locate support and other resources.

## Helping the bereaved family cope

When a loved one dies, the bereaved family needs your emotional support and practical assistance. Although you'll tailor your interventions to meet a family's specific needs, you should keep these general guidelines in mind.

☐ Arrange for staff members to cover for you so that you can focus your energies on helping the bereaved family.

☐ If possible, encourage the family to notify relatives and close friends before the patient dies. This is especially important if only one family member is present. Offer to make phone calls if necessary.

☐ After the patient dies, encourage family members and friends to view the body. This facilitates the grieving process.

☐ Offer to call the hospital chaplain or another member of the clergy and the psychiatric clinical nurse specialist.

☐ Try to provide a quiet, private environment for the family to grieve.

☐ Stay with the family unless they want to be alone. You don't need to say anything—just your presence will be comforting.

☐ Offer family members juice, soda, coffee, or snacks, if possible. They may be too busy thinking about their loss to consider their own needs.

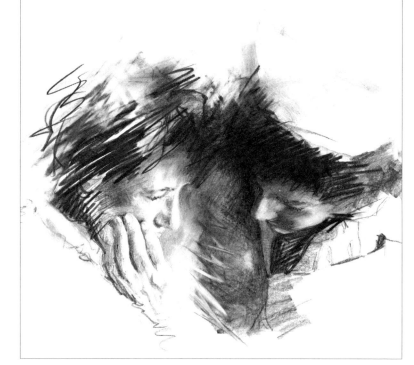

# Evaluation

To determine your patient's acceptance of the loss, observe how he copes. Are his coping mechanisms adaptive or maladaptive? In particular, note any maladaptive reactions, such as unrealistic denial, outbursts of anger, and severe depression or withdrawal.

Consider grieving to be effective if the person deals with his loss in a healthy, positive way. For a dying patient, this might mean that he accepts his death and that he dies at peace and in accordance with his beliefs. For a surviving family member, effective grieving leads to an acceptance of the loss and an ability to move on with his life.

### Requesting a consultation

Depending on the circumstances, you may request a consultation at any point in the nursing process. Usually, you'll assess, intervene, and evaluate the patient before consulting with a psychiatrist or psychiatric clinical nurse specialist.

But in some cases, you'll request a consultation earlier. For example, you should seek a consultation when a patient develops severe psychosocial problems or when patient-staff interactions become severely strained.

### Suggested readings

Barry, P.D. *Psychosocial Nursing Assessment and Intervention,* 2nd ed. Philadelphia: J.B. Lippincott Co., 1989.
Coolican, M., et al. "Helping Survivors Survive," *Nursing89* 19(8):52-57, August 1989.
Deadman, J., et al. "Threat and Loss in Breast Cancer," *Psychological Medicine* 19(3):677-81, August 1989.
*Diagnostic and Statistical Manual of Mental Disorders,* 3rd ed., revised. Washington, D.C.: American Psychiatric Association, 1987.
Gerety, E. "Grieving, Anticipatory Grieving, Dysfunctional Grieving," in *Psychiatric Mental Health Nursing: Application of the Nursing Process.* Edited by McFarland, G.K., and Thomas, M.D. Philadelphia: J.B. Lippincott Co., 1991.
Gorman, L.M., et al. *Psychosocial Nursing Handbook for the Nonpsychiatric Nurse.* Baltimore: Williams & Wilkins Co., 1989.
Kübler-Ross, E. *On Death and Dying.* New York: Macmillan Publishing Co., 1970.
Mian, P. "Sudden Bereavement: Nursing Interventions in the ED," *Critical Care Nurse* 10(1):30-41, January 1990.
Miles, A. "Caring for Families when a Child Dies," *Pediatric Nursing* 16(4):346-49, July-August 1990.
Steele, L.L. "The Death Surround: Factors Influencing the Grief Experience of Survivors," *Oncology Nursing Forum* 17(2):235-41, March-April 1990.
Theut, S., et al. "Resolution of Parental Bereavement after a Perinatal Loss," *Journal of the American Academy of Child and Adolescent Psychiatry* 29(4):521-25, July 1990.
Tom-Johnson, C. "Talking Through Grief," *Nursing Times* 86(1):44-46, January 1990.
Vargas, L.A., et al. "Exploring the Multidimensional Aspects of Grief Reactions," *American Journal of Psychiatry* 146(11):1484-88, November 1989.
Williams, S., and Aguilera, D. "Crisis Intervention," in *Mental Health-Psychiatric Nursing: A Holistic Life-Cycle Approach,* 2nd ed. Edited by Beck, C., et al. St. Louis: C.V. Mosby Co., 1988.
Wilson, H.S., and Kneisl, C.R. *Psychiatric Nursing,* 3rd ed. Menlo Park, Calif.: Addison-Wesley Publishing Co., 1988.

# 8

# SCHIZOPHRENIA AND OTHER PSYCHOTIC DISORDERS

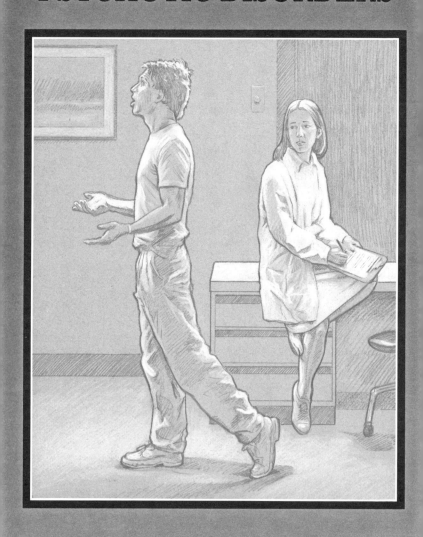

From time to time, you may encounter a patient who seems disconnected from the real world. Perhaps, he lives in a withdrawn cocoonlike state, oblivious to everything around him, or maybe he hears voices.

Chances are such a patient is suffering from some form of psychosis. Characterized by a bizarre personality and a distorted sense of reality, psychosis comes in a variety of forms. And as a nurse, you need to be able to recognize these disorders and give appropriate care to a psychotic patient.

This chapter will help you do that. It discusses psychotic disorders, focusing on the most common one, schizophrenia. The chapter also provides you with important assessment steps, nursing interventions, and evaluation guidelines that you'll need to properly care for a psychotic patient.

# Understanding psychosis

Easy to recognize but difficult to understand, psychosis can occur in acute episodes, chronically, or in a full-blown psychotic illness such as schizophrenia. Although most commonly associated with psychiatric disorders, psychosis usually has organic origins and can be diagnosed through physical and neurologic examinations and laboratory tests. Organic causes of psychosis include neurologic, endocrine, and metabolic disorders; systemic illness; postoperative states; and chemical toxicity and withdrawal.

Psychiatric disorders involving psychosis include schizophrenia, delusional disorder, and other psychotic disorders not elsewhere classified. Psychotic episodes can also occur in mood disorders, such as mania, depression, and manic-depressive illness; and in borderline personality and stress disorders, such as posttraumatic stress disorder. But the leading psychotic disorder remains schizophrenia.

## Schizophrenia

The most common psychotic disorder, schizophrenia affects mood, emotion, thought processes, behavior, and total personality integrity. Psychosis isn't continually present, and symptoms vary greatly from patient to patient. Thus, schizophrenia can be very difficult to diagnose. (See *Criteria for diagnosing schizophrenia,* page 124.)

*Incidence.* Schizophrenia affects about 1% of the population. It usually occurs first in adolescence or early adulthood, but it can also occur in middle and late adulthood. Genetic studies reveal a higher prevalence in people with a family history of schizophrenia and a disproportionately high rate in lower socioeconomic groups. In the United States, the highest incidence occurs in the Northeast. Other studies have shown that schizophrenia occurs in densely populated urban areas twice as often as in sparsely populated rural areas.

*Sociologic concerns.* Before the mid-1950s, most patients with schizophrenia were institutionalized in state psychiatric hospitals. But after the introduction of antipsychotic medications, psychiatric hospitals began releasing patients to their families and community-based programs.

In the 1960s, lawsuits brought against state psychiatric hospitals mandated better care and, combined

# Criteria for diagnosing schizophrenia

To diagnose schizophrenia, a doctor must first rule out organic disorders, schizoaffective disorders, and mood disorders with psychotic features as possible causes. He then uses the following criteria from the *Diagnostic and Statistical Manual of Mental Disorders,* 3rd edition (revised), to confirm his diagnosis:
• in the active phase, one of the following persists for at least 1 week (unless the symptoms are successfully treated):
 —bizarre delusions that the patient's culture would regard as totally implausible, such as thought broadcasting
 —prominent auditory hallucinations of one or more voices
 —at least two of the following: delusions, prominent hallucinations, incoherence or marked loosening of associations, catatonic behavior, or flat or grossly inappropriate affect
• marked decrease in the patient's ability to perform self-care tasks, function at work, and maintain social relationships
• continuous signs of the psychotic disturbance for at least 6 months, during which the patient displays psychotic symptoms of the active phase and possibly symptoms of the prodromal or residual phases. (In the *prodromal phase,* which leads to the active phase, the patient demonstrates a clear deterioration in function; in the *residual phase,* impaired function persists.)
• if the patient has a history of autistic disorder, prominent delusions or hallucinations.

with political concerns about the poor conditions in some state psychiatric hospitals and economic concerns about the cost of long-term hospitalization, led to a nationwide movement to release patients. But

unlike the patients released in the 1950s, most of these patients had no families or support systems, and the community-based programs lacked the funds to help them.

As a result, many psychotic people are now homeless. And even when they are hospitalized, they're typically discharged back onto the streets after a brief stay, with little if any improvement in their condition.

**Types of schizophrenia.** There are four basic classifications of schizophrenia, based on characteristic clinical presentations. These include catatonic type, disorganized type, paranoid type, and undifferentiated type. (See *Understanding types of schizophrenia.*)

**Phases of schizophrenia.** Schizophrenia typically involves three distinct, identifiable phases: prodromal, active, and residual.

*Prodromal phase.* This phase is marked by a notable decline in job or school performance, social relations, or self-care. Manifestations may include an inability to complete assignments, leading to poor work performance or lower grades in school; withdrawal from friends, family, sports, hobbies, or other interests; and inattention to physical appearance, health, or nutrition.

The patient's decline typically has many different aspects and rarely occurs in isolation; his behavioral changes during this prodromal phase are usually associated with other psychiatric disorders, such as depression.

*Active phase.* In this phase, the patient experiences disturbances in his *thought content*—his thoughts, beliefs, and interpretation of events he

# Understanding types of schizophrenia

The *Diagnostic and Statistical Manual of Mental Disorders*, 3rd edition (revised), describes four basic types of schizophrenia.

**Catatonic schizophrenia**
One or more of the following psychomotor disturbances dominate the patient's behavior:
- *stupor* — a diminished response to the environment or a decrease in spontaneous movement and activities
- *negativism* — an apparently motiveless resistance to instructions and attempts to move the patient
- *rigidity* — the maintenance of a fixed posture despite attempts to reposition the patient
- *excitement* — a purposeless increase in motor activity that occurs despite the lack of external stimuli
- *posturing* — the assumption of inappropriate or bizarre stances.

The patient's condition may shift rapidly between stupor and excitement. He may also exhibit mutism (an inability or refusal to speak), stereotypy (repetition of senseless acts or words), mannerisms, and waxy flexibility (the maintenance of whatever body position he is placed in).

**Disorganized schizophrenia**
A doctor won't arrive at this diagnosis until he has ruled out catatonic schizophrenia. The main characteristics of disorganized schizophrenia include incoherence, loosening of association, disorganized behavior, and blunted or grossly inappropriate affect. The patient also may display such abnormal behaviors as marked social withdrawal, grimacing, mannerisms, and hypochondriacal complaints.

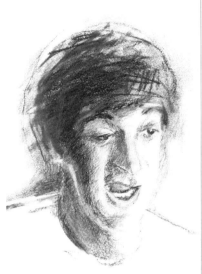

**Paranoid schizophrenia**
If a patient shows none of the signs or symptoms of catatonic or disorganized schizophrenia, he may have this disorder. The paranoid schizophrenic is preoccupied with delusions or frequent auditory hallucinations. Unfocused anxiety, anger, argumentativeness, and violence characterize his behavior. His interactions with others are extremely intense or have a formal, stilted quality.

**Undifferentiated schizophrenia**
Only after ruling out all other types of schizophrenia can the doctor diagnose undifferentiated schizophrenia, which causes prominent hallucinations, delusions, incoherence, or grossly disorganized behavior.

has experienced. The primary disturbance involves *delusions,* which are false, fixed beliefs that cannot be easily changed through reason or experience and that are considered in the patient's societal context to be bizarre, implausible, or fantastically impossible.

A common example of delusion is *thought broadcasting*—the patient's belief that he can telecast thoughts outside of his head or transmit them through telepathic means. Another example is *thought insertion*—the patient's belief that his thoughts aren't his own but rather are being transmitted into his brain by others. In many cases, these delusions take on a persecutory or abusive tone, triggering paranoia.

Another common delusion is *referential thinking*—assigning untoward significance to events, people, or objects. For example, a patient may express referential thinking toward a television or radio broadcast that he thinks is being directed specifically at him.

*Dysfunctional thoughts* involve the disorderly intake and processing of information, and the disorderly expression of ideas. A person's thoughts may be loosely associated, and his speech may flit from topic to topic without any progression or logic. In severe cases, a person's speech may become incomprehensible. Conversely, a patient may have poverty of content; his speech may seem normal, but it conveys little or no coherent information.

Less common types of thought disturbances include neologisms, thought blocking, perseveration, and clang association. *Neologisms* are words the patient coins and endows with a special meaning that only he comprehends. For example, a schizophrenic may refer to any love object as "prattlepie." He may call other patients as well as the pillow he carries "prattlepie."

In *thought blocking*, a patient interrupts his expression of an idea before it's completed. *Perseveration* involves the persistent repetition of words, expressions, or ideas. In *clang association*, a patient chooses

words based on their similar sounds.

Disturbances of perception involve *hallucinations*, in which the mind misinterprets sensory stimuli. In schizophrenia, auditory hallucinations are the most common; the patient typically experiences auditory hallucinations as voices coming from outside his head, often conveying persecutory and self-deprecating messages. Command hallucinations refer to voices directing the patient to perform a specific act—often to harm himself or others.

*Residual phase.* Following the active phase, the residual phase commonly involves many of the same symptoms as the preceding phases. Another characteristic, however, is blunted affect—restricted facial expression and body movement with a congruent mood and monotonous speech—or inappropriate emotional expression.

**Theories on the causes of schizophrenia.** Despite advances in diagnostic technology and psychiatry, relatively little is known about the causes and treatment of schizophrenia. Although current technologic imaging techniques, such as positron-emission tomography (PET) scanning, have shown structural and functional brain changes in people with schizophrenia, the changes remain poorly understood. Over the years, various theories have attempted to explain the cause of schizophrenia.

*Psychological theories.* For years, psychological theories dominated explanations of schizophrenia. These theories hold that schizophrenia is not a disease but rather an adaptation to impaired family relationships.

Working from documents only,

Freud concluded that schizophrenia stemmed from "unconscious homosexuality," which led to an inverted Oedipus complex, in which the patient became attached to his father instead of his mother. In response to Freud's work, Carl Jung and Karl Abraham suggested that the cause was biologically induced, most likely from trauma. Freud countered that the trauma was psychologically — not biologically — induced. The debate continued for many years. Several theories emerged, most of them relating to the time of the causative trauma.

Harry Stack Sullivan, an American psychoanalyst, felt that parent-child conflict (for example, a mother acting in a cold and rejecting manner) was the source of the psychic trauma that caused schizophrenia. In the 1950s, thinking shifted to the double-bind, or mixed-message, theory. This theory held that schizophrenia stemmed from one or both parents' communication to a child that he was both good and bad, both approved of and disapproved of simultaneously.

Although once very popular, these theories lack supportive data — in fact, much new data dispute them — and they do not fit well with current neurobiological findings.

*Neurobiological theories.* Studies in neuroscience have strongly supported the notion that schizophrenia is a disease or possibly many diseases. In 1972, the brains of three schizophrenic patients were autopsied just after death. The studies showed that their brains contained fewer neurons than the brains of normal people; they also revealed diffuse cellular changes.

More recently, computed tomography (CT) scans of living schizophrenics have shown abnormalities in the brain structure of one-third of those examined. These abnormalities included enlarged ventricles, atrophy, and cerebellar abnormalities. Various functional differences have also been measured on EEG, and research conducted at the National Institute of Mental Health with PET scans has shown decreased glucose utilization in the frontal lobes of schizophrenics.

Although a definitive cause for schizophrenia has not been discovered, these studies show promise and have been useful in advancing the knowledge of brain dysfunctions. Much of the current literature continues to distinguish between organic and functional psychosis, but new findings could soon make this distinction obsolete.

*Genetic theories.* The role of genetics in schizophrenia has long been debated. Though the argument has never been settled, available evidence suggests that some link does exist. Among the general population with no known family history of schizophrenia, incidence is about 1%, as compared with 10% in offspring with one schizophrenic parent and 39% in offspring with two schizophrenic parents.

Studies of adopted offspring support this genetic link. In Denmark, children of schizophrenics who were adopted and later examined as adults retained their increased risk of developing the disorder.

Because not all people with an increased risk actually develop schizophrenia, current theories examine the possibility of an acquired predisposition to the disease. According to these theories, predisposition to the disease — rather than the disease itself — may be the inherited trait, as in diabetes, cancer, heart disease, hypertension, and other disorders.

*Other theories.* Current studies are exploring the roles of biochemical alterations, nutritional alterations, and stress in schizophrenia. But to date, no definitive findings have been published.

## Other psychiatric disorders involving psychosis

Several other psychiatric disorders have been linked to psychosis, including mania, major depression, borderline personality disorder, and posttraumatic stress disorder.

**Mania.** A patient experiencing a manic episode exhibits an abnormally exaggerated and persistently elevated or irritable mood. Symptoms of mania include a grandiose sense of self, a significant decrease in sleep, rapid and pressured speech, racing thoughts, distractibility, increased intensity in goal-directed activities, and excessive indulgence in pleasurable activities, such as sexual promiscuity or spending binges beyond the patient's means.

A manic episode can include psychotic delusions or hallucinations (usually auditory) that are mood-congruent, or related to the patient's mood. These delusions or hallucinations contain themes of inflated power, worth, or knowledge. Commonly, the patient claims to have telepathic communication with famous people or religious figures, or even to be such a person. (For instance, a young woman may cling to the delusional belief that she was a waitress at the Last Supper.) Psychotic delusions also can be mood-incongruent, or unrelated to the patient's mood. Examples include delusions of persecution, thought insertion, thought broadcasting, and auditory hallucinations. Catatonia also may occur.

**Major depression.** In a major depressive episode, the patient has a depressed mood marked by reduced interest and pleasure. Such an episode with mood-congruent psychotic features involves delusions or hallucinations (most commonly auditory) containing themes of guilt, self-worthlessness, self-deprecation, disease, or death. The patient also may experience mood-incongruent psychotic episodes and catatonia, as in a manic episode.

**Borderline personality disorder.** This complex, chronic identity disturbance involves instability and lability in behavior, self-image, interpersonal relationships, and mood. Extreme stress may trigger transient psychotic episodes that may or may not require treatment.

**Posttraumatic stress disorder (PTSD).** This incapacitating anxiety disorder affects people who have experienced or witnessed a disturbing event outside the range of normal human experience. The event commonly involves a significant threat to life or physical or emotional integrity. Psychotic features associated with PTSD include recurrent hallucinations, dissociations (flashbacks), and illusions that involve the reliving of the trauma, evoking thoughts and emotions that the person experienced during the original event.

## Organic causes of psychosis

Possible organic causes of psychosis include postoperative states, which can result in postoperative psychosis; chemical abuse; and neurologic disorders. Other organic disorders can also produce signs and symptoms of psychosis. (See *Physical disorders that cause signs of psychosis.*)

***Postoperative psychosis.*** A label commonly given by nonpsychiatric staff members to a patient exhibiting a behavioral change with no readily discernible cause, this psychotic state calls for immediate supportive care and investigation of the underlying cause. Symptoms — abrupt changes in mood or personality, agitation, delusions, and hallucinations — may pose an immediate risk to the patient's medical management, recovery, and even life.

Although stress linked to the threat of loss of life, self-control, or self-identity and fueled by fear and anxiety can precipitate a confusional state, this usually isn't the cause of the psychotic symptoms. In most cases, careful assessment will reveal an underlying organic cause, such as medication intolerance (particularly with anesthetics, analgesics, and steroids) or central nervous system (CNS) depression resulting from cardiopulmonary or infectious complications.

***Chemical abuse.*** Increasingly, you may be caring for patients whose drug abuse is a primary or concomitant focus of hospitalization. Acute intoxication with and withdrawal from many substances can trigger psychosis and violent behavior.

Cocaine or amphetamine abuse may produce drug-induced psychosis. Signs and symptoms may include racing thoughts, pressured speech, psychomotor agitation, hallucinations (visual, auditory, or tactile), paranoid delusions, and violent behavior.

Acute withdrawal from alcohol and barbiturates also can stimulate psychotic episodes similar to those in intoxication and delirium. Psychosis resulting from withdrawal occurs from several days to 2 weeks after the patient has stopped using

## Physical disorders that cause signs of psychosis

The disorders listed below can produce signs and symptoms similar to those of psychosis:
☐ drug toxicity (corticosteroids, digitalis, disulfiram, isoniazid, levodopa, and methyldopa)
☐ endocrine disorders (Addison's disease, Cushing's syndrome, hyperparathyroidism, hypoparathyroidism, and hypothyroidism)
☐ heavy metal poisoning (lead, manganese, mercury, and thallium)
☐ infections (bacterial meningitis, cerebrovascular syphilis, delirium related to cerebral infection, and postencephalitic syndrome)
☐ neurologic disorders (brain tumors, complex partial temporal lobe seizures, degenerative central nervous system diseases, hydrocephalus, and multiple sclerosis)
☐ substance abuse disorders (alcohol intoxication or withdrawal, amphetamine intoxication, barbiturate withdrawal, drug-induced mania, and phencyclidine intoxication)
☐ vitamin deficiencies (niacin, pyridoxine, and thiamine deficiencies and pernicious anemia)
☐ other disorders (atropine psychosis, general paresis, insecticide poisoning, pheochromocytoma, porphyria, Schilder's disease, systemic lupus erythematosus, tubercular meningitis, and Wilson's disease).

the alcohol or barbiturates. Along with psychosis, the patient experiences seizures, disorientation, altered level of consciousness, elevated vital signs, and hyperreflexia.

***Neurologic disorders.*** Various neurologic disorders, resulting from injuries or organic causes, can alter thought processes temporarily or permanently. Identifying an injury-related psychosis is usually easier than pinpointing an organic neurologic cause; this difficulty can lead to erroneously attributing psychosis to a psychiatric disorder.

Neurologic disorders that can cause psychosis include head trauma, brain tumors, vascular lesions (such as infarcts, clots, and hemorrhage), seizure disorders, degenerative brain diseases (such as Alzheimer's and Huntington's diseases), and CNS infections.

New advances in diagnostic technology have made diagnosing organic causes of psychosis easier. Neuropsychological testing by a qualified psychologist can help identify and isolate potential areas of brain malfunction. An EEG, a CT scan, magnetic resonance imaging (MRI), and a PET scan may confirm organic defects in brain structure and functioning.

*Other organic disorders.* Psychosis may accompany other organic illnesses. Suspect an organic cause when the patient experiences an acute onset of altered perception, thought process, or behavior with no history of similar events or when he exhibits impaired consciousness, memory, orientation, perception, or intellectual functioning. In most cases, careful physical and laboratory examination will reveal the causative disorder.

### Challenges in patient care
You may find caring for a psychotic patient extremely challenging. Problems such as noncompliance with therapy, difficulty communicating, withdrawal, and even violent behavior, combined with the chronic nature of the disorder, may arouse in you feelings of frustration, helplessness, anxiety, and maybe even fear.

You may find it particularly distressful to witness the initial onset of schizophrenia in a once-healthy young person, or feel useless when you care for a chronically psychotic patient who shows no improvement despite your best efforts. For some nurses, working with mentally ill patients evokes uncomfortable thoughts of friends or family members with similar illnesses.

A psychotic patient may become isolated from the staff. His strange and sometimes violent behavior, frightened or frightening affect, or bizarre thoughts may alienate you and other staff members.

If you're not sure how to care for a psychotic patient, or you're having difficulty dealing with your own or another staff member's emotions, consult with a psychiatrist or psychiatric clinical nurse specialist. They can teach you techniques for handling psychotic episodes, help you develop an effective care plan for the patient, and help you better understand and cope with your own feelings.

## Assessment

Your goal is to explore the underlying cause of the patient's psychotic episode. Only then can you identify and implement effective interventions.

### Obtaining a patient history
Obtain a detailed history from the patient or, if necessary, from his family members or others well-acquainted with him. If the patient's medical records are available, review them for information that concerns his normal and abnormal behavioral patterns. Obtain the

names of any current outpatient caregivers treating the patient for his psychiatric illness.

For the patient with a known mental illness, investigate what exacerbated his illness. If the health history fails to reveal any evidence of a preexisting psychiatric illness, explore possible organic causes for the psychosis.

### *Identifying events that trigger symptoms.* Investigate the patient's history for any events that could trigger the onset of psychotic symptoms. Medication noncompliance and stress are two likely possibilities.

Ask the patient which antipsychotic medication he's taking, what the prescribed dosage is to control symptoms, and when he last took the drug. If this information isn't available, consult with a doctor for a serum drug level measurement, which may yield important information on the patient's use of the medication.

If you detect noncompliance, ask the patient why he failed to take the prescribed drug. Does he experience any adverse effects when he takes the drug? Does he sometimes forget whether he has taken the drug? Does he have enough money to buy the drug?

Explore whether any stressful events may have triggered the psychotic episode. (Even if he fully complies with his medication regimen, a psychotic patient may experience a relapse in response to severe physical or emotional stressors.) Ask the patient whether he has recently been ill or sustained any injury. Has he experienced any recent losses, such as the death of a loved one or loss of income, housing, therapists, or relationships? Is this the anniversary of a significant loss?

### Assessing behavioral characteristics
Determine the patient's recent behavioral patterns. Look for signs of disturbed thoughts, altered perceptions, altered communication, altered affect, altered motor activity, and impaired intellectual and social functioning.

*Disturbed thoughts.* Psychosis may produce delusional thoughts that the patient finds either distressing (egodystonic) or acceptable and of no concern (ego-syntonic). Ask the patient what kinds of thoughts he has been having, whether he's comforted or frightened by these thoughts, and if he's planning to take any action based on them.

*Altered perceptions.* Sensory alterations, especially prominent in the early phases of schizophrenia, can range from blunting or enhancement (most common) to full-blown hallucinations. Determine whether the patient is experiencing auditory enhancement or hallucinations. Does background noise seem conspicuously louder, as if someone has turned up the volume? Does he hear voices from outside his head? Is he comfortable with what the voices are saying? Does he trust the voices? Are the voices directing him to do things (command hallucinations), such as hurt himself or others? Keep in mind that the patient is at greater risk of harming himself or others if he trusts the voices.

Is the patient experiencing visual enhancement or hallucinations? Do colors appear brighter than before? Does he see visions? If so, what are they?

Keep in mind that visual hallucinations may include any distortion of visual stimuli or visions not seen by others. In schizophrenia, visual

CHECKLIST

## Recognizing psychotic communication

A psychotic patient often has difficulty communicating and may have one or more of the speech dysfunctions listed below.

☐ *Tangential speech*. The patient shifts from topic to topic. Each new topic shares only an oblique connection with the previous one.

☐ *Loose association*. The patient speaks in jumbled statements, with one topic having no logical connection to the previous topic. For instance, when you ask the patient how you can improve his care, he may respond, "Improve? Can't improve. Can't prove a thing. I'm in this jail, and you can't prove I did anything."

☐ *Circumstantial speech*. The patient eventually returns to his original point, but only after moving from topic to topic, adding unnecessary details throughout.

☐ *Echolalia*. The patient repeats (or echoes) words spoken to him—possibly in an attempt to synthesize what he has heard.

☐ *Thought blocking*. The patient cuts off the flow of his speech before finishing his idea and then can't recall the blocked thought.

☐ *Perseveration*. The patient repeats the same word or phrase over and over.

☐ *Clang association*. The patient uses rhyming or alliteration. For instance, he might say, "Clean the sink, think, rink, fink..."

☐ *Word salad*. The patient uses a meaningless jumble of words.

☐ *Concrete thinking and speech*. The patient can't make the switch from concrete concepts to abstractions. For example, if you tell him to "clean his plate" at dinner, he'll take you literally and immediately get up to wash it.

hallucinations rarely occur without auditory hallucinations. But if they do occur alone, evaluate the patient for an organic cause of the psychosis.

Is the patient experiencing any enhancement or distortions in the sense of touch? Although rare in schizophrenia, this can occur and may be caused by psychomotor seizure activity.

What about altered senses of smell and taste? An altered sense of smell suggests another cause of the psychosis, such as psychomotor seizure activity.

If an altered sense of taste occurs without auditory hallucinations, evaluate the patient for drug intoxication, drug or alcohol withdrawal, psychomotor seizure activity, or CNS infection.

*Altered communication.* Evaluate the patient for altered speech patterns typical of psychosis. (See *Recognizing psychotic communication.*) When talking with him, note the sequence or pattern of the ideas or thoughts he expresses. Do his responses relate well to your questions? Are his associations among ideas sound or loose? Can he organize the information he's communicating? Do his ideas have logical connections? Can he understand abstract concepts, or does he exhibit concrete thinking? (For instance, if you ask, "Do you feel OK?" does he feel something and then respond, "Yes, I do"?) Does he add a lot of unnecessary information while trying to get to the point of his response? What about the words he chooses? Is he using rhyme or alliteration? Is he repeating words or phrases over and over? Does he seem to have a meaning other than the generally accepted one for the words he's using?

***Altered affect.*** Evaluate the patient's emotional response to others. Does he appear distant, impersonal, or unable to reciprocate feelings with another person? Can he express a wide range of emotions? Does he exhibit normal fluctuations in mood or emotional lability? Do his emotions seem appropriate for the situation? Can he communicate his emotions through facial or other nonverbal clues?

Keep in mind that exaggerated emotional responses typically don't occur in schizophrenia beyond the disorder's early phases. Expect to see inappropriate or flattened affect, and withdrawal occasionally punctuated by rapid mood changes.

***Altered motor activity.*** Observe the patient's activity level. Is he restless, or very quiet and almost motionless? Although psychotic disturbances may produce psychomotor agitation (for example, pacing in response to hallucinations or delusions), more common motor responses involve slowed reactions or reduced movements or activity. In extreme cases, the patient may exhibit no conscious awareness of his environment (catatonic stupor), with rigid body movements or waxy flexibility (the maintenance of whatever body position he's placed in).

***Impaired intellectual and social functioning.*** Assess the patient's intellectual and social functioning in relation to the way he functioned before the onset of his psychotic disorder. Look for impaired work or school performance, and disinterest in interpersonal relationships and

self-care. As the psychosis progresses, expect to see increased withdrawal from society as bombardment from both external and internal stimuli preempts the patient's concern with other people, work, and self-care.

## Identifying an impending psychotic crisis

As mentioned earlier, stressful situations can precipitate a psychotic episode in a person predisposed to schizophrenia or other forms of psychosis. In a high-risk patient, watch for early signs of an impending psychotic episode, including:
• abrupt or gradual changes in mental status or thought processes, as indicated by altered speech patterns
• auditory hallucinations, possibly accompanied by other sensory disturbances
• changes in affect, either inappropriate (for example, smiling and laughing while describing the loss of a loved one) or restricted (displaying a less-than-normal level of emotion)
• altered thought form (for example, thought insertion, broadcasting, or blocking)
• fixed, paranoid delusions.

## Assessing the risk of injury

The psychotic patient is at the greatest risk of harming himself and others when he's actively hallucinating. Command hallucinations may instruct him to kill or hurt himself or others. Sensory enhancement and the inability to process information may frighten him and cause him to strike out at others or harm himself. The inability to connect thoughts logically or to synthesize information correctly may lead him to make poor judgments about hazards in his environment, causing him to disregard obvious dangers.

Be sure to assess the psychotic patient's potential for violence and risk of injuring himself and others, particularly when he's actively hallucinating.

# Intervention

To select the most effective interventions for a psychotic patient, you first need to identify the underlying cause of the psychotic episode. If the cause is organic, the patient must receive treatment to resolve the symptoms. The patient with uncontrolled schizophrenia needs evaluation and readjustment of his medication regimen. If stressors have precipitated a psychotic event in the controlled schizophrenic patient, you need to identify and deal with these stressors.

But your immediate priority in a psychotic episode should be to intervene to prevent injury to the patient and others. After ensuring safety, you can perform other interventions directed at resolving the underlying cause.

### Ensuring safety

During a psychotic episode, regardless of its underlying cause, you may need to provide aggressive antipsychotic drug therapy and apply restraints to protect the patient and others from harm. Keep in mind that you should use restraints only as a last resort. (See *Preventing an assault* for more information on how to deal with a potentially violent patient.)

Because of their rapid onset, I.V. neuroleptics and benzodiazepines are the drugs of choice for treating a patient experiencing a psychotic episode. However, drug action may

not occur for up to 30 minutes after administration. For a psychotic patient deemed at imminent risk of violence either to himself or others, restraints are necessary until the drugs take effect.

In most cases, you'll use leather restraints for a violent psychotic patient. Keep in mind, however, that most states have laws mandating that you use the least restrictive devices possible when restraining a patient, to prevent injury.

After restraining the patient, monitor him closely. Every 15 minutes, assess comfort, body position, behavior, and airway patency. At least every hour, ask the patient how he feels and whether the restraints are causing him any pain. Also assess nutrition, warmth, elimination, and circulation and perfusion status of the restrained limbs. Assess vital signs every 2 hours.

Unless a medical emergency occurs, never remove the restraints without a psychiatrist's order. When removing restraints, take them off gradually so that you can evaluate the patient's impulse control.

If you've determined that the patient is at an increased risk for suicide, you'll need to institute suicide precautions.

### Resolving underlying organic causes

Tailor your interventions aimed at resolving the underlying cause of psychosis specifically to the cause. For example, when treating alcohol-induced psychosis, you need to know the current amount of alcohol use. Because the patient usually isn't a reliable source for this information, the doctor may estimate the patient's current tolerance by administering test doses of barbiturates or benzodiazepines and by observing their effects. He'll pre-

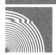

## Preventing an assault

When dealing with an aggressive and potentially violent psychotic patient, take the following measures to help avoid a crisis:

• Avoid approaching a potentially violent patient alone. Summon other staff members or security personnel when necessary.

• Leave the patient's door open when you're providing care to allow you to make a quick exit or call for help.

• Stay more than an arm's-length away from the patient.

• Be prepared to move away quickly. A violent patient can strike out suddenly.

• Look for and, if possible, remove every object in the patient's immediate environment that he could possibly use as a weapon, including eating utensils, writing instruments, lamps, trays, and other equipment.

• Administer any prescribed antianxiety or antipsychotic medication early on during the aggressive episode, before the patient becomes violent. If necessary, restrain him first. But avoid restraints unless you sense a clear and present danger.

• If you must restrain the patient, make sure you have enough help available. Ideally, you'll need five people — one at each limb and the fifth to control the patient's head.

• Never remove restraints (except in a medical emergency) without the permission of the psychiatric consultant.

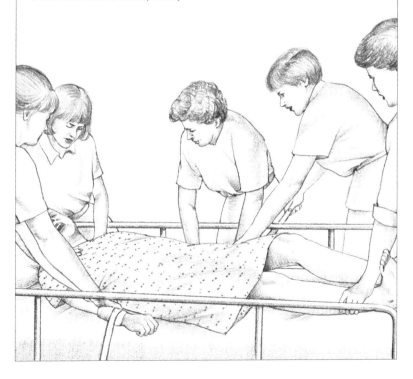

scribe the estimated dosage, then gradually decrease the dosage over several days. During the withdrawal period, monitor vital signs frequently and take seizure precautions.

Keep in mind, however, that you may not be able to address the underlying cause in some patients. For example, treatment for neurologically induced psychosis usually is limited to supportive interventions.

## Establishing a therapeutic relationship
Effective interventions depend on developing a therapeutic relationship with the patient. First, you need to demonstrate a caring attitude to gain the patient's trust. A trusting nurse-patient relationship may help avert the need for restraints and can promote the patient's compliance with the prescribed treatment regimen.

When approaching a psychotic patient, remain calm and maintain a certain distance between you and him. When talking to the patient, use simple, jargon-free phrases. Never argue with the patient about his delusions or hallucinations or deny that he's experiencing them. Rather, help orient him to reality by stating simply that you don't perceive the hallucinations. For instance, if the patient states, "There are bricks on my bed," you might say, "I don't see any bricks on the bed, only sheets and your pillow," then change the subject. You also may find setting limits and repeating explanations and instructions helpful in therapeutic communication.

When performing any procedure, explain every step before you do it, allowing the patient time to process the information before you proceed. You may allow him to touch the equipment you'll be using to help reduce his fear. If he's still afraid, postpone the procedure until later, if possible.

Because a psychotic patient can't think abstractly, be sure to use words and phrases that are easily understood and unambiguous. Choose your words carefully because the patient will tend to take everything you say literally. For instance, if you tell a patient that a scheduled test will be done "right on the floor," he may become frightened, thinking he'll actually have to lie on the floor for the procedure.

After your relationship with the patient seems secure, focus your interventions on helping him express his real feelings and ideas, make decisions comfortably, accept pleasurable experiences, and control his anxiety. Once you've developed an effective care plan for the patient, share the information with other staff members to ensure consistent care.

## Administering antipsychotic drugs
To treat hallucinations, delusions, aggressive or violent behavior, and thought disorders associated with psychosis, expect to administer antipsychotic (sometimes called neuroleptic) drugs. These drugs bind with dopamine receptor sites in the brain, controlling hallucinations, delusions, and disordered thinking.

Effective antipsychotic drug therapy can reduce symptoms, decrease the length of hospital stays, and minimize the need for rehospitalization. Concomitant benzodiazepine therapy (commonly with lorazepam or diazepam) may help control acute psychosis associated with anxiety, aggression, or violence.

The doctor commonly will prescribe an antipsychotic drug to treat acute psychotic thinking associated with organic causes. He'll avoid these drugs in acute psychosis attributed to drug intoxication or withdrawal because they may obscure the diagnosis.

You'll provide antipsychotic drug therapy in three stages: acute management, stabilization, and maintenance.

***Types of antipsychotic drugs.*** Recognize that antipsychotic drugs are categorized by potency. High-potency drugs include fluphenazine hydrochloride (Prolixin), haloperidol (Haldol), thiothixene (Navane), and trifluoperazine (Stelazine). Intermediate-potency drugs include loxapine succinate (Loxitane), molindone (Moban), and perphenazine (Trilafon). Low-potency agents include chlorpromazine (Thorazine) and thioridazine (Mellaril).

***Adverse drug effects.*** Be aware of the three primary types of adverse effects associated with antipsychotic drugs: sedative, anticholinergic, and extrapyramidal. Also note that specific adverse effects vary with drug potency. High-potency antipsychotics are minimally sedative and minimally anticholinergic but carry a high risk of extrapyramidal adverse effects. Intermediate-potency agents carry a moderate risk of sedative, anticholinergic, and extrapyramidal adverse effects. Although highly sedative and anticholinergic, low-potency antipsychotics carry a low risk of extrapyramidal adverse effects.

When selecting an antipsychotic drug for a patient, the doctor weighs the desired effects against the risk of adverse effects. He then prescribes the lowest effective dosage to minimize the adverse effects. He also may prescribe a long-acting injectable form of the antipsychotic drug, which may minimize the risk of adverse effects, or concomitant anticholinergic drug therapy to specifically reduce extrapyramidal effects.

During drug therapy, monitor the patient for adverse effects. Observe him particularly for the most common extrapyramidal effects — dystonia, parkinsonism, and akathisia — and for neuroleptic malignant syndrome and hypotension.

*Dystonia.* Characterized by anguished tonic contractions of muscles in the neck, mouth, and tongue, dystonia is commonly misdiagnosed as a psychotic symptom. It usually affects young males, typically within the first few days of treatment. If you note dystonia, notify the doctor, who will order an anticholinergic agent (usually diphenhydramine or benztropine) administered I.M. or I.V. to provide rapid relief.

*Parkinsonism.* Drug-induced parkinsonism is marked by slowed movements, muscle rigidity, shuffling or propulsive gait, stooped posture, flat facial affect, tremors, and drooling. These effects may occur from 1 week to several months after initiation of drug therapy. Drugs prescribed to reverse or prevent this syndrome include benztropine, trihexyphenidyl, and amantadine.

*Akathisia.* Characterized by restlessness, pacing, and an inability to rest or sit still, akathisia is another antipsychotic drug-induced extrapyramidal effect. Propranolol has proven effective in relieving this complication.

*Neuroleptic malignant syndrome (NMS).* Occurring in 0.5% to 1% of people receiving antipsychotic drugs, this rare and life-threatening complication of antipsychotic drug therapy involves fever, muscle rigidity, and an altered level of consciousness. Onset of symptoms typically occurs from 1 to 3 days after initiation of drug therapy, but it can occur anytime within several hours to several months after the start of therapy. If you detect NMS, act quickly to institute supportive and symptom-targeted interventions, which may include medications to counter muscle rigidity and hyperthermia. Be sure to assess vital signs and mental status frequently.

*Hypotension.* Most commonly associated with low-potency antipsychotic drug therapy, hypotension necessitates prompt intervention. Place the patient in a supine position and give him I.V. fluids. As ordered, administer an alpha-adrenergic agonist, such as norepinephrine or metaraminol; a mixed alpha- and beta-adrenergic drug, such as epinephrine; or a beta-adrenergic drug, such as isoproterenol.

# Evaluation

Evaluate the patient's behavior based on the outcome criteria for each identified problem. For instance, determine whether his ability to think and reason has returned to the same level as before his psychotic episode. Also evaluate the effectiveness of drug therapy in controlling symptoms. If the patient's psychotic state is linked to a chronic psychiatric cause and he needs continuing care in an outpatient setting, determine which setting he should go to. Does he know where the facility is? Does he understand the importance of keeping his scheduled appointments and taking his prescribed medication?

You may find it difficult to determine how successfully the patient will adapt to an unsupervised setting. His distorted thinking will tend to impair his ability to comply with long-term drug therapy and seek help if symptoms recur.

## Requesting a consultation

Depending on the circumstances, you may request a consultation at any point. You may assess the patient and perform some interventions before consulting with a psychiatrist or psychiatric clinical nurse specialist. Or you may request a consultation earlier. For instance, you should request a consultation if the patient has, or may have, a psychiatric diagnosis. Also, if your patient becomes suicidal, have him evaluated immediately by a psychiatric clinical nurse specialist or a psychiatrist.

When evaluating the need for consultation, consider the following questions:
• Do those caring for the patient have enough information about the patient's disorder?
• Do caregivers disagree about the treatment plan?
• Do staff members attempt to avoid caring for the patient?
• Are communication and interventions proving effective?

Dealing with a psychotic patient can present various problems if you're not experienced in psychiatric care. The patient may evoke in you feelings of fear (especially when he is agitated or violent) and anxiety (from your unfamiliarity with the bizarre symptoms associated with psychotic disorders). Another problem is the limited amount of time you have to deal effectively with a psychotic patient on a busy unit. In many cases, the time needed just isn't available.

You can consult with a psychiatrist or a psychiatric clinical nurse specialist if you need more information on how to deal effectively with psychotic patients. These professionals can help develop a care plan that addresses both the patient's and the nursing staff's needs, taking into consideration time constraints and other conditions. They also can offer suggestions to help you and other staff members recognize and deal with your feelings.

## Suggested readings

*Diagnostic and Statistical Manual of Mental Disorders,* 3rd ed., revised. Washington, D.C.: American Psychiatric Association, 1987.

Gay, P. *Freud: A Life for Our Time.* New York: W.W. Norton & Co., 1988.

Gomez, G.E., and Gomez, E.A. "Chronic Schizophrenia: The Major Mental Health Problem of the Century," *Perspectives in Psychiatric Care* 27(1):7-9, 1991.

Groves, J.E., and Manschreck, T.C. "Psychotic Patients," in *Massachusetts*

*General Hospital Handbook of General Hospital Psychiatry.* Edited by Hackett, T.P., and Cassem, N.H. Chicago: Year Book Medical Pubs., 1987.

Harper, G. "Focal Inpatient Treatment Planning," *Journal of the American Academy of Child and Adolescent Psychiatry* 28(1):31-37, January 1989.

Hatfield, A.B. "The National Alliance for the Mentally Ill: A Decade Later," *Community Mental Health Journal* 27(2):95-103, 1991.

Hatfield, A.B. "Patients' Accounts of Stress and Coping in Schizophrenia," *Hospital and Community Psychiatry* 40(11):1141-44, November 1989.

Jenike, M.A. *Geriatric Psychiatry and Psychopharmacology: A Clinical Approach.* Chicago: Year Book Medical Pubs., 1989.

Jung, C.G. "On the Psychogenesis of Schizophrenia," in *The Basic Writings of C.G. Jung.* Edited by De Laszlo, V.S. New York: The Modern Library, 1959.

Miller, E. "Clinical Thinking in Diagnosis-Based Nursing Practice," in *How to Make Nursing Diagnosis Work.* Edited by Miller, E. Norwalk, Conn.: Appleton & Lange, 1989.

Murray, G.B. "Confusion, Delirium, and Dementia," in *Massachusetts General Hospital Handbook of General Hospital Psychiatry.* Edited by Hackett, T.P., and Cassem, N.H. Chicago: Year Book Medical Pubs., 1987.

Stuart, G.W., and Sundeen, S.J. *Principles and Practice of Psychiatric Nursing,* 4th ed. St. Louis: Mosby-Year Book, Inc., 1991.

# 9

# EATING DISORDERS AND OBESITY

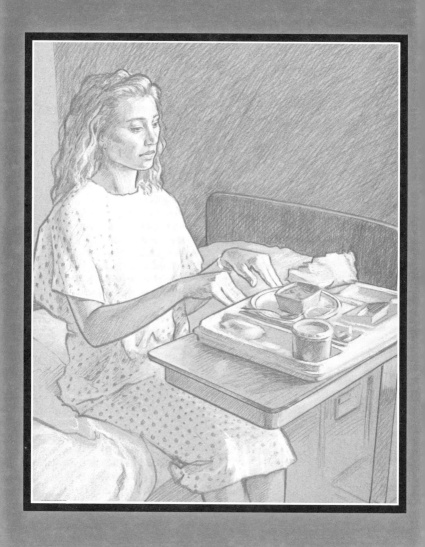

In our weight-obsessed society, where the mass media constantly bombard us with visions of the "ideal" body — a slim, sleek, perfectly proportioned figure for women and a lean, taut, muscular physique for men — more and more people feel compelled to take whatever steps are necessary to conform to this image.

Consequently, unsound quick weight-loss and fitness gimmicks have proliferated, making many entrepreneurs very rich but leaving millions of consumers frustrated and dissatisfied. Binge eating, crash dieting, and general dissatisfaction with one's body image are common and, in and of themselves, not considered abnormal. But when these behaviors interfere significantly with a person's health, they're considered an eating disorder and require treatment.

In the United States, eating disorders affect about 1.2 million adolescent and adult females. The incidence among males is considerably lower. The overall incidence has remained fixed at about 5% of the population for the past 5 years. Although typically associated with adolescent and college-age females, in recent years eating disorders have begun to occur more frequently among women in their 30s and 40s, particularly highly ambitious, success-oriented professionals in stressful positions.

This chapter explores two common eating disorders: anorexia nervosa and bulimia nervosa. Although obesity is not considered an eating disorder, it's included in the chapter because of its profound physical and psychosocial ramifications. For all three of these problems, you'll find a thorough explanation, including appropriate nursing assessment, intervention, and evaluation.

# Understanding eating disorders

Eating disorders present no typical clinical picture. At first glance, a person with an eating disorder may appear healthy and well adjusted. Rarely will you see overt signs, such as emaciation. As a result, identifying an eating disorder is often difficult.

## Types of eating disorders

Defined as entities or syndromes rather than diseases with a common cause, course, and pathology, eating disorders are classified into two major categories: anorexia nervosa and bulimia nervosa.

The American Psychiatric Association's *Diagnostic and Statistical Manual of Mental Disorders,* 3rd edition (revised), describes anorexia nervosa as a gross disturbance in eating behavior and sets specific criteria for its diagnosis. (See *Criteria for diagnosing anorexia nervosa,* page 142.)

A patient with anorexia nervosa controls weight solely by self-starvation (restricting food intake) and excessive compulsive exercise. In contrast, a patient with bulimia nervosa controls weight through self-starvation alternating with episodic binge eating and purging — using laxatives, diuretics, or self-induced vomiting to prevent weight gain. (See *Criteria for diagnosing bulimia nervosa,* page 143.) A person who exhibits anorexia and binge-purge behavior has both anorexia nervosa and bulimia nervosa.

## Causes of eating disorders

Various theories attempt to explain

## Criteria for diagnosing anorexia nervosa

To diagnose anorexia nervosa, a doctor will use the criteria listed in the *Diagnostic and Statistical Manual of Mental Disorders,* 3rd edition (revised), which include:
• refusal to maintain minimal normal body weight
• an intense fear of gaining weight or becoming fat, even though the patient is already underweight
• a distorted body image — for example, the patient "feels fat" even when emaciated
• in women, the absence of at least three consecutive menstrual cycles when they should have occurred.

why eating disorders develop. Possible causes include biological factors, family influences, and psychological factors.

**Biological factors.** Four possible biological factors can play a part in causing eating disorders or can be triggered by an eating disorder and in turn exacerbate it. They include hypothalamic dysfunction, excessive cortisol secretion, low serotonin levels, and endogenous endorphins.

*Hypothalamic dysfunction.* Amenorrhea secondary to self-starvation and excessive exercise disrupts hypothalamic function. This initially causes a decrease in appetite stimulation and eventually leads to total appetite suppression.

*Excessive cortisol secretion.* A person with an eating disorder secretes excessive amounts of cortisol, which act on the hypothalamus, decreasing appetite stimulation. Excessive cortisol secretion also may cause de-

pression, which may further diminish appetite and lead to decreased food consumption.

*Low serotonin levels.* Serotonin (5-HT) in the brain helps regulate eating, mood, and impulse control. Low 5-HT levels may cause a depressed mood and a decreased appetite. Tryptophan, a metabolite of carbohydrate consumption, is converted to 5-HT. This may explain why a person temporarily feels elated during a food binge or during rapid carbohydrate consumption. Some antidepressant medications also raise 5-HT levels in the brain, lifting the depression.

*Endogenous endorphins.* Current research is exploring the role that endogenous endorphins (opiate receptors) play in the binge-purge cycle. The kappa opioid receptor in the brain may become overstimulated in people with eating disorders, resulting in binge-purge behavior. Naltrexone, a long-acting opioid antagonist, has been shown to stop the binge-purge cycle.

**Family influences.** A healthy parent-child relationship provides opportunities for the child to develop as an individual, promoting independence and autonomy in preparation for adulthood. In contrast, dysfunctional families discourage independence, promoting feelings of powerlessness and helplessness — feelings that can set the stage for an eating disorder. When caring for a person with an eating disorder, your knowledge of family dynamics may help you assess the underlying cause and plan effective care.

The noted family therapist Salvador Minuchin has identified four characteristics commonly present in the family of an anorexic or a bulimic person: enmeshment, overprotectiveness, rigidity, and lack of conflict resolution.

*Enmeshment.* Extreme intensity in family interaction and communication among family members results in blurred boundaries between the role of the parent and the role of the child. The child loses her sense of self-identity and has trouble differentiating herself from the family.

*Overprotectiveness.* The parents' excessive concern for the child's welfare retards her development of autonomy, competence, and interests outside the safety of the family, commonly leading to social isolation.

*Rigidity and lack of conflict resolution.* The family's inflexibility in adapting to change and dealing with interpersonal conflict impairs its members' ability to solve problems and cope with stress.

**Psychological factors.** Hilde Bruch, a noted psychiatrist, relates anorexic and bulimic behavior to underlying deficits in a person's sense of self-identity and autonomy. She theorizes that primarily through unconscious mechanisms, the person maintains childlike behavior, has difficulty making decisions, and avoids responsibility. Through self-starvation, the person strives to achieve a childlike appearance and avoid becoming an adult.

**Immediate causes.** A crisis situation commonly precipitates anorexic or bulimic behavior. The most common crises involve some kind of loss. Examples include the death or serious illness of a family member or friend, marital conflict or divorce, loss of a friendship, unemployment, or moving away from a familiar place.

## Criteria for diagnosing bulimia nervosa

To diagnose bulimia nervosa, a doctor will use the following criteria from the *Diagnostic and Statistical Manual of Mental Disorders,* 3rd edition (revised):
• recurrent episodes of binge eating (at least two a week for 3 months or more)
• a feeling of lack of control over eating during these binges
• prevention of weight gain through self-induced vomiting, strict dieting, vigorous exercise, or use of laxatives or diuretics
• obsession with body shape and weight.

### Challenges in patient care
Eating disorders pose a unique challenge to your nursing skills. You may find long-term management in an outpatient setting both frustrating and rewarding. Be aware that treatment is lengthy and complex, and that the patient may require hospitalization during treatment.

A major challenge to the nurse stems from the fact that anorexic and some bulimic patients typically deny the problem and rarely seek treatment. The patient tries to hide her problem, feeling scared and helpless over what's happening to her. Although she may want to resume normal eating habits, she commonly believes that she can't do it on her own. In many cases, she feels that she's the only one with this problem and fears what others will think and how they'll respond to her if they find out about it.

The patient's mistrust of health care professionals and need for control commonly make a therapeutic relationship difficult to achieve.

# Anorexia nervosa

Anorexia nervosa is characterized by a distorted body image. Regardless of her actual weight, the patient views herself as "fat" and continually strives for an "ideal" body through self-starvation and excessive exercising.

Although the patient typically retains an interest in food — in fact, is obsessed by it — her need for control overrides her desire to eat. Limiting food intake provides this sense of control. The patient's obsession manifests itself in such behaviors as concealing or hoarding food, throwing food away, or cutting food into small pieces. She also may exhibit compulsive behavior, such as arranging food in particular patterns on the plate or eating only a particular type, texture, or color of food.

The anorexic patient is also commonly obsessed with exercise and maintains a high energy level even as her body weight decreases. To her, exercise is a ritual and a compulsion, and she experiences a great deal of anxiety if she can't exercise after eating.

## Assessment
In many cases, a patient's family member or friend will alert you to a possible eating disorder. Confirming anorexia, however, requires a careful health history, a thorough physical assessment, and diagnostic tests.

*Patient history.* Begin with a complete medical history to rule out other disorders, such as cancer and tuberculosis, that produce symptoms mimicking those of anorexia nervosa. Investigate such complaints as frequent abdominal bloating, ulcer-like pain, and constipation. Also explore any past or present substance abuse and any current indications of depression.

Through careful history taking, you may detect behavioral clues pointing to anorexia. Such clues can include erratic eating patterns, frequent or constant dieting, excessive exercise, interpersonal or family problems, substance abuse, and psychological problems such as depression.

*Eating and exercise patterns.* Explore past and present eating patterns, any history of dieting, the types of diets the patient has tried, successes and failures with these diets, and the patient's average weight over the past 3 to 5 years. (See *Assessing eating patterns.*) Also find out about exercising, including the type, frequency, and duration of exercise. An anorexic patient may exercise often and vigorously, even immediately after eating.

*Family history.* When obtaining a family history, check for eating disorders among female relatives. Note that sisters and daughters of those with anorexia nervosa have a higher incidence of the disorder than the general population. Also check for any history of depression in immediate family members.

*Sexual and reproductive history.* Take a sexual history during the interview. The patient may express fear of or disinterest in intimate sexual relationships, or dissatisfaction with her sexual relationships.

Determine the patient's menstrual history. In many anorexic patients, amenorrhea develops up to a year before significant weight loss occurs. The characteristic menstrual pattern involves progressively shorter cycles progressing to irregular menses, then to amenorrhea. Be aware that in an anorexic adolescent, menarche may be delayed and the menstrual cycle will be irregular during the first year after menarche.

*Social patterns.* Explore the patient's social interactions. The anorexic patient commonly avoids socializing with peers and may be withdrawn and isolated. At school or work, she may be a high achiever, even a perfectionist. At home, she may be viewed as a "model" child or wife.

*Self-concept.* Also assess the patient's self-concept. An anorexic person integrates the highly desirable (to her) characteristic of thinness into her self-concept. This leaves her vulnerable to such problems as low self-esteem and poor self-image if she can't reach and maintain her perceived ideal weight.

*Assessment tools.* You may use an assessment tool, such as the eating attitudes test, to help explore the patient's feelings about food and eating and to monitor treatment progress. (See *Eating attitudes test,* page 146.) Keep in mind that the eating attitudes test isn't useful in monitoring behavior, the duration of the eating disorder, vomiting frequency, or body image distortions.

Another useful assessment tool is a food journal, in which the patient records the types and amounts of foods she eats, when she eats, and her feelings about eating and exercise. You can discuss this information with the patient to help pinpoint the nature of the problem.

**Physical assessment.** Begin your physical assessment by weighing

### Assessing eating patterns

When assessing a patient's eating patterns, look closely at the following:
- types and amounts of foods eaten
- times when eating occurs
- length of time spent eating
- where eating occurs – for example, in the kitchen or dining room, at a restaurant, in front of an open refrigerator or a TV
- how meals are eaten – for example, alone, with companions, on the run, or in the car
- emotional states that trigger eating – for example, boredom, depression, loneliness, anger, frustration, or stress
- activities that stimulate eating – for example, social events.

the patient. Consider a body weight decrease of 15% or more a medical emergency requiring hospitalization.

Also note any of the following signs and symptoms: loss of breast tissue or regression of breast development, visible bony prominences, hypotension with bradycardia, lanugo (fine, downy hair) on the back and arms, dry skin, brittle hair, hypothermia, abdominal distention from bloating or constipation, slowed reflex responses, and muscle weakness and atrophy.

**Diagnostic tests.** Evaluate the results of all ordered diagnostic tests. Routine blood work for a patient with suspected anorexia includes a complete blood count (CBC), an electrolyte profile, an erythrocyte sedimentation rate (ESR), a prolactin level, and a thyroid profile. Results suggesting anorexia may include iron deficiency anemia on the CBC, a normal electrolyte profile, decreased ESR and prolactin level, and

# Eating attitudes test

The eating attitudes test lets you evaluate a patient with a suspected eating disorder.

Name: _____

Date: _____

| | A Always | B Very often | C Often | D Sometimes | E Rarely | F Never |
|---|---|---|---|---|---|---|
| I'm terrified of becoming overweight. | | | | | | |
| I don't eat when I'm hungry. | | | | | | |
| I find myself preoccupied with food. | | | | | | |
| I've gone on eating binges that make me feel like I may not be able to stop. | | | | | | |
| I cut my food into small pieces. | | | | | | |
| I'm aware of the calorie content of the food I eat. | | | | | | |
| I particularly avoid foods that have a high carbohydrate content (such as bread, potatoes, and rice) | | | | | | |
| Other people would prefer me to eat more. | | | | | | |
| I feel extremely guilty after eating. | | | | | | |
| I'm preoccupied with a desire to be thinner. | | | | | | |
| I think about burning up calories when I exercise. | | | | | | |
| Other people think I'm too thin. | | | | | | |
| I'm preoccupied with the thought of having fat on my body. | | | | | | |
| I take longer than others to eat my meals. | | | | | | |
| I avoid foods that contain sugar. | | | | | | |
| I eat diet foods. | | | | | | |
| Food controls my life. | | | | | | |
| I display self-control around food. | | | | | | |
| Others pressure me to eat. | | | | | | |
| I give too much time and thought to food. | | | | | | |
| I feel uncomfortable after eating sweets. | | | | | | |
| I engage in dieting behavior. | | | | | | |
| I like my stomach to be empty. | | | | | | |
| I enjoy trying rich new foods. | | | | | | |
| I have the impulse to vomit after meals. | | | | | | |
| I make myself vomit after eating. | | | | | | |

From Button, E.J., & Whitehouse, A. (1981). Subclinical anorexia nervosa. *Psychosomatic Medicine*, 11, 509-516.

a normal thyroid profile except for a decreased triiodothyronine ($T_3$) value, which is directly related to slowed metabolism from limited food intake.

Also evaluate any other diagnostic tests, which may include an electrocardiogram (ECG), skull and chest X-rays, and the Mantoux test for tuberculosis. Negative results help rule out other medical disorders that can mimic anorexia nervosa.

## Intervention

Treating anorexia nervosa is a complex and lengthy process involving aggressive medical management, psychotherapy, and nutritional counseling. It's best accomplished by a treatment team consisting of a doctor and nurse familiar with eating disorders, a nutritionist, and a psychotherapist or psychiatric clinical nurse specialist.

Treatment may be provided on an outpatient basis or may require hospitalization to correct serious medical complications or nutritional deficits, as in the case of a patient who has lost considerable weight and needs a structured environment. (See *When should an anorexic patient be hospitalized?*)

***Weight maintenance.*** For an outpatient, focus your interventions on maintaining or increasing body weight and preventing substantial weight loss (15% or more of total body weight). You can accomplish this by establishing a target weight (typically, at least 90% of the patient's ideal body weight) and contracting with the patient to eat sufficient amounts to achieve this target weight. Especially at the beginning of therapy, the patient will hover right around this target weight without gaining any more weight. Use a standard weight chart

## When should an anorexic patient be hospitalized?

An anorexic patient needs hospitalization if she:
☐ rapidly loses 15% or more of her total body weight
☐ develops persistent bradycardia (50 beats/minute or less)
☐ becomes hypotensive (a systolic reading of 90 mm Hg or lower)
☐ becomes hypothermic (a core body temperature of 97° F [36° C] or lower)
☐ develops medical complications
☐ expresses suicidal thoughts
☐ persistently sabotages or disrupts her outpatient treatment
☐ adamantly denies her need for help.

to establish the patient's ideal weight range. (See *Standard weight chart,* page 148.) To monitor her progress and condition, perform weekly weigh-ins along with temperature, blood pressure, and heart rate assessments.

For a hospitalized patient, aim for an average weight gain of about 1 lb/week. Provide one-to-one supervision during meals and for 1 hour afterward.

Whenever possible, allow the patient to maintain some control over the types and amounts of food she eats. Explain to the patient that she'll lose this privilege if she fails to comply with her contract or if a life-threatening complication develops. Unless absolutely necessary, avoid forced tube feedings and total parenteral nutrition in the hospitalized patient because they'll make her feel that she has no control.

***Psychotherapy.*** Individual psychotherapy is aimed at recognizing and changing behavior. In the course of

## Standard weight chart

The weight chart below, developed by the United States Departments of Agriculture and Health and Human Services, reflects the current thinking that people can safely add more weight as they age. Because people of the same height have different body types, you'll find the ideal weight given as a range. Higher weights in each category typically apply to men and lower weights to women.

| HEIGHT (without shoes) | IDEAL WEIGHT FROM AGE 19 TO 34 | IDEAL WEIGHT AT AGE 35 AND OVER |
|---|---|---|
| 5'0" | 97-128 lb | 108-138 lb |
| 5'1" | 101-132 lb | 111-143 lb |
| 5'2" | 104-137 lb | 115-148 lb |
| 5'3" | 107-141 lb | 119-152 lb |
| 5'4" | 111-146 lb | 122-157 lb |
| 5'5" | 114-150 lb | 126-162 lb |
| 5'6" | 118-155 lb | 130-167 lb |
| 5'7" | 121-160 lb | 134-172 lb |
| 5'8" | 125-164 lb | 138-178 lb |
| 5'9" | 129-169 lb | 142-183 lb |
| 5'10" | 132-174 lb | 146-188 lb |
| 5'11" | 136-179 lb | 151-194 lb |
| 6'0" | 140-184 lb | 155-199 lb |
| 6'1" | 144-189 lb | 159-205 lb |
| 6'2" | 148-195 lb | 164-210 lb |
| 6'3" | 152-200 lb | 168-216 lb |
| 6'4" | 156-205 lb | 173-222 lb |
| 6'5" | 160-211 lb | 177-228 lb |
| 6'6" | 164-216 lb | 182-234 lb |

the therapy, the patient explores her pursuit of thinness, her need to maintain control, and her self-concept. Ideally, she will come to understand her relationship with food and learn how she uses it as a substitute for other behavior, will learn to relinquish some control without losing her individuality, and will gain self-confidence and increased self-esteem.

Group therapy allows the patient to share information in a setting that can reduce her sense of shame and her perceived need for secrecy. It also allows for reality testing with peers, which can help dispel unrealistic beliefs and expectations common in anorexic patients. Group therapy also may help her decrease social isolation, promote social skills, and develop more effective communication techniques.

Family therapy can help take the pressure off the patient, who may feel solely responsible for the problem. In effective therapy, family members learn more effective communication and problem-solving techniques.

By developing a trusting relationship with the patient and her family, you can reinforce the progress made in psychotherapy and provide support during ongoing therapy.

*Patient teaching.* Aim your patient teaching at providing information on proper nutrition and weight maintenance. As the patient comes to trust the treatment team, she'll become more open to suggestions about maintaining adequate weight without the fear of becoming overweight. As necessary, provide information on adolescent anorexic behavior to the patient's family. (See *Caring for adolescents with eating disorders.*) Also, refer the patient and her family to an available

## Caring for adolescents with eating disorders

When caring for an adolescent with anorexia or bulimia, keep in mind that the following developmental factors may influence the progression of the disorder and affect your approach.

☐ The patient may be struggling to assert her independence, amplifying her fear of control and making family therapy difficult.

☐ If the patient is afraid or unsure of her emerging sexuality, she may try to remain a child by starving herself, halting breast development, menstruation, and other signs of sexual maturation.

☐ The patient may readily fall prey to peer pressure and to media influences that hold up thinness as the ideal.

☐ Normal adolescent rebellion may hinder your ability to form a therapeutic relationship with the patient.

☐ Adolescents tend to be healthy, which masks the subtle physiologic clues that point to an eating disorder.

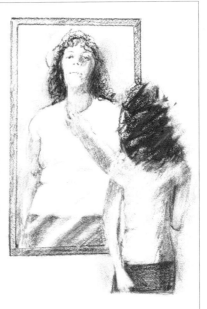

support group and encourage their participation.

## Evaluation

Determine the effectiveness of treatment for an anorexic patient by evaluating her weight gain or by assessing how well she has maintained the negotiated target weight. Also assess the patient's psychological status, noting signs of improved self-esteem and self-image.

*Requesting a consultation.* Depending on the circumstances, you may request a consultation at any point. You may assess the patient and perform some interventions before consulting with a psychiatrist or psychiatric clinical nurse specialist.

Or you may request a consultation earlier. For instance, you should seek a psychiatric consultation whenever you suspect depression in an anorexic patient. Depression may lead to suicidal tendencies, requiring immediate psychiatric intervention. You should also seek a consultation if you detect signs and symptoms of anorexia in a previously undiagnosed patient.

# Bulimia nervosa

The predominant characteristic in bulimia nervosa is binge eating that alternates with fasting or purging.

Although frequent weight fluctuations may occur, weight loss usually isn't as severe as it is in anorexia nervosa.

Although bulimia can affect people of any age and either sex, the typical patient is female, white, single, and college-educated. Rarely an only child, she usually comes from a dysfunctional family and can be from any socioeconomic class. The patient commonly struggles alone between 4 to 6 years before seeking treatment.

The eating binges, characterized by rapid consumption of high-calorie foods, usually occur at least twice a week, during periods of stress or anxiety. The foods the person consumes are typically sweet, with a texture that allows rapid eating without much chewing. The person usually binges surreptitiously and stops only when prompted by abdominal discomfort, social interruption, sleep, or self-induced vomiting, known as purging.

The binge episode actually represents an altered state of consciousness, which the patient typically remembers as a blurred experience. She feels elated during the binge but later has self-deprecating thoughts and may be depressed.

Binging, purging, and laxative, diuretic, or emetic use all serve as vehicles for psychological expression. Binging helps regulate mood, affect, impulse expression, self-nurturing, and oppositionality (acting out, defiance). Purging releases tension, especially aggression, and alleviates the guilt associated with binging. It also serves as self-punishment for the binge. On a conscious level, purging relieves abdominal discomfort and either ends the binge or allows it to continue. The use of laxatives, diuretics, or emetics gives the bulimic patient the power to control her weight and relieve her guilt.

## Assessment

Explore your patient's bulimia with a focused patient history and physical assessment. Also, evaluate pertinent laboratory test results for characteristic findings.

*Patient history.* Begin the history by obtaining information on the patient's history of dieting; weight fluctuations and average weight over the past 3 to 5 years; laxative, emetic, and diuretic use; and elimination patterns.

Ask about any history of substance abuse. The bulimic patient may use such drugs as alcohol, amphetamines, and cocaine to help maintain weight control or lose weight.

*Emotional and mental status.* Ask whether the patient experiences episodes of depression. If so, how long do they last? How do they make her feel? Are they precipitated by any particular events? Do they occur during a particular season of the year?

Major depression affects approximately 50% of bulimic patients. So during the interview, observe the patient for signs of depression. Does she appear sad? Does she avoid direct eye contact? Note her personal hygiene and grooming. When speaking, does she sound tired, sigh or speak slowly, or have difficulty continuing conversations?

Does she experience sleep disturbances, such as difficulty falling or staying asleep, early morning awakening, or sleeping longer hours yet continually feeling fatigued? What about difficulty concentrating or deteriorating work or school performance?

Also assess for suicidal ideation. Ask the patient what she sees herself doing 1 month, several months, and 1 year from now. Has she ever felt like hurting herself? Does she feel this way now? If so, does she have a plan for accomplishing this? These questions may elicit important information. Any indication or suspicion of depression, with or without suicidal ideation, necessitates immediate consultation with a psychiatric clinical nurse specialist or a psychiatrist.

Does the patient frequently experience feelings of guilt, frustration, and anxiety? Does she find it difficult to express her feelings, especially anger?

*Family history.* Determine if the patient has a family history of bulimia, anorexia, or obesity. (Many bulimic patients have obese parents.) Also check for any family history of depression or substance abuse. Ask the patient about any major conflicts that exist within her family unit.

*Sexual and reproductive history.* When exploring the patient's sexual and reproductive history, note especially any reports of unsatisfying sexual relationships or promiscuity, both of which are common in bulimic patients. Like the anorexic patient, the bulimic patient may experience irregular menses or amenorrhea.

*Social history.* Explore how the patient views herself and her social ability. If possible, contrast the patient's views with those of another family member. In many cases, a bulimic patient feels socially insecure and fears a loss of control within her environment, whereas friends and family members perceive her as socially competent, in-

dependent, strong, and in control.

***Physical assessment.*** Begin your physical assessment by weighing the patient. The bulimic patient tends to be either within the normal weight range for her height, age, and body frame type, or only slightly to moderately above or below this range.

In most cases, your assessment won't reveal any physical findings indicating bulimia nervosa. You may, however, detect signs that point to excessive self-induced vomiting, such as enlarged, nontender parotid glands; hoarseness; throat irritation; calluses on the knuckles (Russel's sign); and dental caries and dental erosion (especially behind the front teeth).

Severe vomiting may produce hemoptysis, conjunctival hemorrhage, and even small, broken blood vessels on the cheeks. Rectal irritation and, in more severe cases, atonic colon may point to chronic laxative abuse.

***Laboratory tests.*** Evaluate the results of all ordered laboratory tests, beginning with serum electrolyte levels. Excessive vomiting and laxative, diuretic, or emetic abuse can cause electrolyte imbalances (most commonly, sodium and potassium alterations), possibly leading to dehydration, acute renal dysfunction, cardiac arrhythmias, or even cardiac arrest.

Because chronic hypokalemia adversely affects the kidneys' ability to excrete waste and the heart's electrical conductivity, pay particular attention to the serum potassium level. Report results below 2.8 mEq/liter. Keep in mind that the risk for potentially fatal cardiac arrhythmias increases as the serum potassium level decreases.

## Antidepressant drugs for patients with bulimia

The chart below lists therapeutic doses and blood levels for drugs used to treat depression in patients with bulimia.

| DRUG | THERAPEUTIC DOSE (mg) | THERAPEUTIC BLOOD LEVEL ($\mu$g/ml) |
|---|---|---|
| amitriptyline (Elavil) | 100 to 200 | 100 to 200 |
| amoxapine (Asendin) | 200 to 300 | 150 to 500 |
| desipramine (Norpramin) | 50 to 250 | 100 to 250 |
| imipramine (Tofranil) | 75 to 250 | 150 to 300 |
| nortriptyline (Pamelor) | 75 to 125 | 50 to 150 |
| trazodone (Desyrel) | 150 to 200 | 800 to 1,600 |

If you suspect renal dysfunction, consult with the doctor about a 24-hour urine collection to evaluate total volume and creatinine clearance. This can reveal renal dysfunction before abnormal blood urea nitrogen and serum creatinine levels can be detected in the blood.

Also evaluate urinalysis results for protein and ketone bodies, which may point to fasting. Note increased urine specific gravity, possibly indicating dehydration, or decreased specific gravity, which may result from the patient water loading to give the impression of weight gain.

### Intervention

As with anorexia nervosa, treatment of bulimia nervosa aims to prevent medical complications and provide psychotherapy and nutritional counseling. During therapy, you'll need to monitor laboratory test results, evaluate the effectiveness and adverse effects of drug therapy, identify possible symptoms of depression or substance abuse, and provide emotional support to the pa-

tient and her family. You should also offer positive reinforcement for any progress the patient makes during psychotherapy.

*Pharmacologic therapy.* As ordered, administer antidepressant medications to treat the depression commonly associated with bulimia nervosa. Commonly prescribed drugs include trazodone and such tricyclic antidepressants as amitriptyline, amoxapine, desipramine, imipramine, and nortriptyline. (See *Antidepressant drugs for patients with bulimia.*) Obtain a baseline ECG before starting drug therapy, and repeat the test periodically during therapy, as ordered.

Monitor the effectiveness of therapy by evaluating the patient's clinical response to the medication, tolerance of adverse effects, and blood drug levels. Expect to see improvement within 2 to 5 weeks after initiating therapy. Watch for and report any adverse effects, which may include dry mouth, constipation, orthostatic hypotension, palpitations, tachycardia, blurred vision, and urine retention.

If hypokalemia causes cardiac arrhythmias, expect to administer po tassium supplements. For mild hypokalemia, you may give 20 mEq of potassium chloride orally once or twice daily until serum potassium levels return to normal. Expect to monitor the patient's serum potassium levels closely until they reach the desired range.

*Psychotherapy.* Refer the bulimic patient for psychotherapy. Individual psychotherapy focuses on challenging the patient's false beliefs and teaching her acceptable ways to deal with her anger and frustration. Effective psychotherapy should help her understand the motivations that underlie her behavior and teach her strategies for controlling her impulses. If the patient has a substance abuse problem, you may need to refer her to a drug rehabilitation program.

In group therapy, food journals are shared with the other patients and their progress is monitored. Through shared experience, the bulimic patient learns that others also battle depression and substance abuse, which may help reduce her feelings of isolation. Sharing can also help the patient learn effective strategies for overcoming these difficulties.

Family therapy offers support as well as strategies for improved family system functioning.

*Patient teaching.* Teach the patient about the hazards of binging, purging, and fasting. Also explain the risks of laxative, emetic, and diuretic abuse. As appropriate, provide assertiveness training and help her develop a realistic and positive self-concept.

### Evaluation
Characterized by their addictive tendencies, patients with bulimia nervosa commonly are more disturbed psychologically than patients with anorexia nervosa. Major depression (often with suicidal ideation), mixed substance abuse, and impulse domination behaviors (for example, shoplifting, self-mutilation, and promiscuity) give the bulimic patient a poor prognosis for a full recovery.

Understand that treatment of bulimia nervosa, like treatment of anorexia nervosa, is a slow process. Several years may pass before you see significant improvement in the patient's condition. When evaluating the effectiveness of treatment, look for gradual resumption of normal eating patterns with no fasting, binging, purging, or laxative, diuretic, or emetic abuse.

Also look for a lifting of the patient's depression, with initial improvement shortly after onset of therapy and continued improvement occurring gradually over the course of the ongoing therapy.

# Obesity

Generally defined as an excess of body fat at least 20% above the ideal weight for a person's age and height, obesity affects a large number of people in the United States. Obesity can be classified as mild, moderate, or severe (morbid). (See *Classifying obesity,* page 154.) The past 20 years have seen a significant rise in childhood and adolescent obesity, which predisposes an individual to adult obesity.

Obesity is a leading cause of hypertension, orthopedic problems,

## Classifying obesity

Whether your patient has mild, moderate, or severe (morbid) obesity depends on how far his weight exceeds the ideal weight for a person of his height and age.
☐ Mild obesity: 20% to 40% above ideal weight
☐ Moderate obesity: 40% to 100% above ideal weight
☐ Severe obesity: more than 100% above ideal weight.

and diabetes. Morbid obesity carries more health risks than either mild obesity or moderate obesity, and it can result in gout, certain types of cancer, and unexplained sudden death.

Obese people or those vulnerable to obesity are generally less active physically than people of normal weight. Morbid obesity leads to decreased physical activity because the excess body weight causes stress on bones and connective tissue, shortness of breath, and decreased cardiac functioning.

Obesity also may contribute to sleep difficulties. Morbid obesity is a major characteristic of pickwickian syndrome — a hypoventilation syndrome caused by intermittent nighttime airway obstruction that produces sleep apnea and hypoxia, interrupting the sleep cycle as the person awakens to resume normal ventilation. This happens repeatedly during sleep and results in daytime somnolence. The combination of obesity plus the sleep-induced relaxation of the pharyngeal muscle probably produces the intermittent airway obstruction. These apneic episodes can produce life-threaten-

ing cardiac arrhythmias.

Along with its physiologic risks, obesity also carries significant psychological ramifications. An obese adult commonly has low self-esteem and a poor self-image, and may be nonassertive and angry. In an obese adolescent, these problems may be magnified because an adolescent may tend to tie body image even more closely to self-concept. Socially, obesity is viewed as unacceptable, and obese people often suffer insults and discrimination, further contributing to their feelings of anger, shame, and low self-esteem.

Even normal-weight adults who suffered childhood obesity commonly report lingering anger and resentment directed at their parents — especially their mothers — for having made them diet and restrict their food intake. These people are also prone to such psychological problems as low self-esteem and nonassertiveness.

### Causes
Obesity results from excessive caloric intake and inadequate energy expenditure. Various factors and theories have been identified in attempts to explain why this occurs.

*Eating behavior.* Obviously, excessive food intake is a major cause of obesity. Unfortunately, eating behavior is not yet completely understood. Appetite is controlled by specific areas of the hypothalamus — a feeding center and a satiety center. Signals sent from the feeding center to the cerebral cortex stimulate hunger.

To prevent overeating, the satiety center sends inhibiting impulses to the feeding center. The satiety center is stimulated by increased plasma glucose levels or insulin following a meal. Meal-induced gastric distention also acts to stimulate the satiety center. These are known as *internal cues* that regulate eating behavior.

Unfortunately, *external cues*, such as taste and smell, tend to dominate eating behavior in obese people as well as people of normal weight. Controlling these external cues is the goal of behavior modification therapy.

**Familial and genetic factors.** Obesity seems to have a familial tendency, but the role of genetics is unclear. A child of one obese parent has a 40% risk of being obese; a child of two obese parents, a 70% risk.

The genetic influences are difficult to pinpoint because of the social and cultural factors associated with food. Food is commonly equated with love, and cultural differences account for different food preferences. In some cultures, obesity is held in high regard.

In one verified genetic type of childhood obesity, known as *juvenile-onset obesity,* the child is born at a normal body weight, but his weight increases rapidly with aging because of accelerated fat cell production. Normally, during the first 2 years of life, fat cell production accelerates and then levels off. Production again accelerates just before puberty, then levels off again. In juvenile-onset obesity, fat cell production continues to accelerate throughout childhood and puberty. The child has up to five times the number of fat cells as a normal-weight child.

Successful weight loss in these patients requires a reduction in the number of fat cells — an extremely difficult proposition.

**Body type.** A person's general body type plays a role in his predisposition to obesity. Humans have three basic body types: ectomorphic, mesomorphic, and endomorphic. (See *Identifying body types,* page 156.) Ectomorphs have thin, lean bodies with relatively little muscle mass. Mesomorphs have "athletic" builds with average amounts of muscle mass. Endomorphs have increased body fat and are most prone to obesity.

**Medical disorders.** Although obesity isn't caused by any medical disorder, certain disorders may contribute to it. These include insulinoma, hypothyroidism, Cushing's disease, and hypothalamic disorders.

**Set point theory.** According to the set point theory, a preset amount of consumed food is expended as energy, and the rest is stored as fat. Through a feedback mechanism involving the hypothalamus and some unknown substance produced by or dissolved in fat, food intake is regulated to maintain a biologically predetermined level of fat stored in adipose tissue.

This mechanism serves as a sensor to increase the amount of energy storage. This may explain why some people remain thin regardless of the amount of food they consume, whereas others find it difficult to lose weight or to maintain weight loss after dieting.

Until recently, childhood obesity was commonly blamed on the parents, especially the mother. Obese children were thought to have been overfed or started on solid food too early in life. Parents were scolded by pediatricians for overfeeding their children and making them fat. Now, the set point theory suggests that infants are born with a preset level of energy expenditure.

## Identifying body types

Use the illustrations below to help you identify your patient's body type.

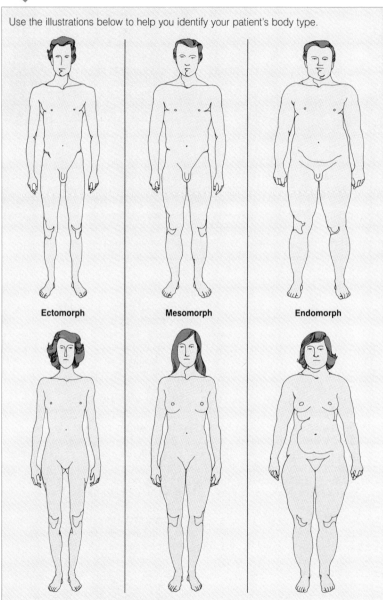

Ectomorph          Mesomorph          Endomorph

*Enzyme deficiency.* Another theory suggests that a deficiency of the enzyme adipose tissue lipoprotein lipase (ATLPL) causes the body to store more triglyceride (pure fat) in adipose tissue.

## Assessment

Explore the extent of your patient's obesity, as well as the underlying causes, through a focused patient history and physical assessment.

*Patient history.* When assessing the obese patient, explore his perceptions of food and eating. Does he eat when he's upset, anxious, or worried? Does he associate food with having fun or being loved? Has he always had a weight problem, or is the weight gain a recent development? If a recent development, was it associated with any particular life event?

Explore the patient's family history. Are other family members obese? Do they share the same dietary habits as the patient? What role did food play in his family when he was growing up? Was he always required to clean his plate as a child? Does he still feel guilty about not finishing all his food?

Assess his normal food intake. How many meals does he eat a day? How much does he eat at one time? Does he snack between meals? Does he eat out at restaurants frequently?

Also explore elimination patterns. Does he experience constipation often? Does he use laxatives routinely?

Ask about any physical complaints that he links to his obesity, such as shortness of breath or sleeping problems. For a female patient, ask about any reproductive dysfunction, such as failure to ovulate or menstrual irregularities.

Finally, explore any prior history of substance abuse and assess the patient's potential for drug abuse before drug therapy.

*Physical assessment.* Although height and weight charts are the most commonly used assessment tool in obesity, they're not the most effective means of assessing obesity. Two other methods are more useful: the body mass index (BMI) and skinfold thickness measurements.

To determine a patient's BMI, take his body weight in kilograms and divide it by his height in meters squared. A BMI of 40 or more indicates morbid obesity.

Use skinfold thickness measurements to determine a patient's total body fat content. With calipers, measure skinfold thickness at three specific body sites: the triceps, suprailium, and thigh in women; and the chest, abdomen, and thigh in men. Take three measurements at each site and average them, then add the three average measurements together and compare the result to a standard body fat percentage chart that lists acceptable skinfold thickness measurements for sex and age-groups.

When assessing a child or an adolescent, observe for signs that suggest he might be vulnerable to obesity. These signs include excessive weight for age, early sexual maturity (including early menarche in girls), advanced bone age, and excessive muscle mass.

## Intervention

Treating weight problems typically requires some combination of diet and exercise programs, pharmacologic therapy, surgical intervention, and psychotherapy. Any underlying mental health problems that influence the patient's eating behaviors, such as depression or anxiety, and any physical problems caused by obesity must be identified and addressed.

***Diet and exercise.*** The goal of diet and exercise programs for weight reduction is to provide fewer calories than the body needs to produce the energy required for the exercise done. Simply stated, to lose weight, the person must burn up more calories than he takes in.

Ensure that your patient's prescribed diet provides adequate amounts of all four food groups as well as adequate vitamins and minerals to prevent malnutrition. Ideally, the best diet is one that promotes slow, steady weight loss, with a variety of food choices to promote compliance.

Be aware that a patient 40 lb or more over his ideal body weight may need to lose large amounts of weight rapidly. This can be accomplished only through severe caloric restrictions known as very-low-calorie diets (VLCDs). These diets, which include liquid, protein-sparing diets, provide 400 to 800 kcal/day and 45 to 70 g/day of high-quality protein from egg or milk-based sources. The patient mixes the powder with water and takes a "meal" three to five times daily.

VLCDs work by inducing ketosis, suppressing appetite, and producing diuresis. Monitor a patient on a VLCD for such adverse effects as postural hypotension, constipation, halitosis, muscle cramping, reversible hair loss, and gouty attacks (rare). In a female patient, assess for irregular menstrual patterns.

Ensure that the patient receives weekly medical supervision during the diet's course. Specific monitoring should include biweekly electro-lyte studies to detect low potassium and calcium levels, which can precipitate dangerous cardiac arrhythmias; a weekly ECG to assess for any cardiac conduction abnormalities; and periodic 24-hour urine collection for creatinine clearance to assess lean muscle mass loss.

Be aware that diet therapy in children and adolescents can pose problems. Restrictive dieting during the growth years may lead to major nutritional deficits.

Ensure that the patient's prescribed exercise program fits his needs and physical capabilities. Reevaluate the program routinely as his physical capabilities improve, and suggest modifications. To promote the patient's compliance with the program, explain that regular exercise accelerates metabolism, diminishes appetite stimulation, and reduces body fat while increasing lean muscle mass. Also point out that exercise has a positive effect on mood and cardiopulmonary function.

***Pharmacologic therapy.*** As ordered, administer the prescribed drug. Under medical supervision, anorexic (appetite-suppressant) agents may be used for short-term, rapid weight loss. However, the potential for addiction, habituation, and generalized drug abuse limits the usefulness of these drugs. (See *Drug therapy for obesity* for information on drugs that you may be administering.)

***Surgery.*** Although generalized weight loss diminishes adipose tissue somewhat proportionately throughout the body, it doesn't always produce the desired cosmetic effects. Currently, no proven technique can eliminate adipose tissue in specific body areas. Liposuction is increasingly used to "spot" reduce fat from the thighs, hips, and buttocks. However, this procedure is expensive and not without surgical risks. Besides posing a risk of infection, fat removal is hindered by nerve endings and blood vessels in surrounding tissue.

For a morbidly obese patient who needs to lose a large amount of weight rapidly, the doctor may recommend surgical intervention, such as gastroplasty (vertical and horizontal band stapling), a jejunoileal shunt (small-bowel bypass), or insertion of a gastric bubble.

*Gastroplasty.* Commonly termed "stomach stapling," this is the least risky and most commonly performed surgical procedure for weight loss. Gastroplasty limits food intake by delaying gastric emptying and providing a small gastric reservoir so that the patient feels full after having just a small meal. Among the advantages of this procedure is that it can be reversed, if so desired.

*Jejunoileal shunt.* Also known as gastric bypass, this effective but risky procedure is performed only on select people who've repeatedly failed at weight-loss attempts despite careful medical management. In this surgery, the surgeon sews a row of sutures to separate the fundus from the body of the stomach. Then he fastens a loop of the jejunum to the fundus, leaving an opening for food passage.

With only about 15% of the stomach working (85% of the stomach is bypassed), the patient feels satisfied with much smaller portions of food. Because of the high risk of postoperative mortality, this procedure is contraindicated in people over age 50 and people who are psychologically unstable.

Possible life-threatening postoperative complications of a jejunoileal

## Drug therapy for obesity

Several drugs can help treat obesity, including amphetamines, benzocaine, bulk fillers, and phenylpropanolamine.

### Amphetamines and amphetamine-like agents
Prescription drugs such as dextroamphetamine (Dexedrine), fenfluramine (Pondimin), and phendimetrazine (Trimstat) suppress the appetite by acting on certain brain centers. These drugs may keep the patient's appetite under control for a week or slightly longer; after that, he may develop a tolerance to the drug.

### Benzocaine
Ayds and other brands of this over-the-counter local anesthetic deaden the tastebuds. As a result, the patient may not enjoy food as much and may eat less.

### Bulk fillers
Fiber-Trim and other over-the-counter bulk fillers absorb water in the stomach and expand to produce a sense of fullness, decreasing the appetite. However, they may paradoxically increase the appetite in some people.

### Phenylpropanolamine
This over-the-counter drug acts like amphetamines and is used only for short-term weight control. Brands include Acutrim and Dexatrim.

shunt include wound infection, thromboembolism, cirrhosis, kidney and liver failure, and electrolyte imbalances. When caring for a candidate for this procedure, make sure he fully understands the risks and possible complications, and arrange for a complete psychological evaluation. Explain that abdominal pain, diarrhea, and vomiting will likely occur for up to 1 year after surgery.

*Gastric bubble.* Another surgical treatment for morbid obesity involves insertion of a gastric bubble. In this procedure, the doctor inserts a 3″ diameter durable balloon through a flexible tube into the patient's stomach, then inflates it. The inflated balloon reduces stomach volume, limiting food intake.

*Psychotherapy.* Behavior modification therapy is based on the premise that both normal-weight and obese people respond to similar external cues associated with eating behavior. Such cues include food taste, smell, visual attractiveness, and abundance, and ease in obtaining food. Effective behavior modification alters the person's responses to these cues. For instance, if a person who usually snacks in the evening while watching TV substitutes walking or riding a bike for TV watching, he's less likely to eat extra food.

For a patient undergoing psychotherapy, give positive feedback for successful behavior modification. This can help enhance his self-esteem and encourage him to continue to comply with treatment.

Building the patient's self-esteem is critical to a successful weight-reduction program. To help, refer the patient to available support groups as needed.

**Evaluation**

Evaluate the effectiveness of the patient's weight-reduction program based on his success at losing weight and maintaining the weight loss over time. Outcome criteria vary, depending on the program. For example, with a liquid, protein-sparing VLCD, expect to see rapid, significant weight loss over a 3- to 6-week period with no medical complications. With continued weight reduction, also look for a resolution of any health problem related to obesity, such as insulin resistance, hyperproteinemia, hypertension, airway obstruction, and sleep disorders.

---

**Suggested readings**

Andersen, T., and Larsen, V. "Dietary Outcomes in Obese Patients Treated with a Gastroplasty Program," *American Journal of Clinical Nutrition* 50(6):1328-40, December 1989.

Blundell, J.E. "Appetite Disturbance and the Problems of Overweight," *Drugs* 39(Suppl 3):1-19, 1990.

Clark, K.L., et al, eds. *Evaluation and Management of Eating Disorders: Anorexia, Bulimia, and Obesity.* Champaign, Ill.: Human Kinetics Pubs., 1988.

Comerci, G.D. "Medical Complications of Anorexia Nervosa and Bulimia Nervosa," *Medical Clinics of North America* 74(5):1293-1310, September 1990.

*Diagnostic and Statistical Manual of Mental Disorders,* 3rd ed., revised. Washington, D.C.: American Psychiatric Association, 1987.

Frankle, R.T., and Yang, M. *Obesity and Weight Control: The Health Professional's Guide to Understanding and Treatment.* Rockville, Md.: Aspen Pubs., Inc., 1987.

Garfinkel, P.E., et al. "Eating Disorders: Implications for the 1990s," *Canadian Journal of Psychiatry* 32(7):624-31, October 1987.

Garrow, J.S. *Obesity and Related Diseases.* New York: Churchill Livingstone, 1988.

Giannini, A.J., et al. "Anorexia and Bulimia," *American Family Physician* 41(4):1169-76, April 1990.

Grana, A.S., et al. "Personality Profiles of the Morbidly Obese," *Journal of Clinical Psychology* 45(5, Mono Suppl):762-65, September 1989.

King, M.B. "Eating Disorders in General Practice," *Journal of the Royal Society of Medicine* 83(4):229-32, April 1990.

Kirschenbaum, D.S., and Johnson, W.G. *Treating Childhood and Adolescent Obesity.* New York: Pergamon Press, 1987.

Laraia, M.J., and Stuart, G.W. "Bulimia: A Review of Nutritional and Health Behaviors," *Journal of Child and Adolescent Psychiatric Mental Health Nursing* 3(3):91-97, July-September 1990.

Lerman, R.H., and Cave, D.R. "Medical and Surgical Management of Obesity," *Advances in Internal Medicine* 34:127-63, 1989.

Palmer, T. "Anorexia Nervosa, Bulimia Nervosa: Causal Theories and Treatment," *Nurse Practitioner* 15(4):12-21, April 1990.

# 10

# CHILD, SPOUSE, AND ELDER ABUSE

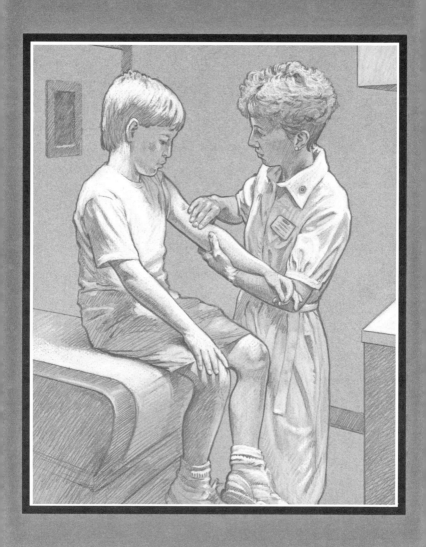

In the United States, an estimated 6 million people, including children and elderly people, are beaten, raped, or neglected every year. An estimated 25% to 30% of all women are victimized sexually before reaching adulthood. To make matters worse, many of these crimes go unreported because the victims are too ashamed or frightened to call the police or seek medical attention.

Abuse crosses all social, racial, ethnic, and religious barriers. But you can identify people and families at risk if you know what risk factors and warning signs to look for. This is where your special nursing knowledge and skills come into play. Besides knowing how to recognize abuse, you'll need to know what physical and psychological interventions to take. And because we're only beginning to understand the devastating aftereffects of abuse, you'll also need to constantly update your skills to help patients cope and recover.

This chapter begins with an overview of abuse and then moves on to cover child, spouse, and elder abuse and rape in detail. Within each section, you'll find key assessment steps, important nursing interventions — including legal interventions that can help protect the victim — and evaluation techniques you can use to give your abused patient the best possible care.

---

# Understanding abuse

How can you tell if a patient has been abused? It's not always easy, but understanding the different types of abuse will help you identify these patients so that you can start

dealing with their problems right away.

## Types of abuse

Abuse is categorized in two general ways: by the type of victim (child, spouse or sexual partner, or elder) and by the method of abuse (physical abuse, sexual abuse, emotional abuse, or neglect). Any type of abuse can also be called domestic abuse if both the abuser and the victim are members of the same family.

*Physical abuse* is an assault involving bodily contact or injury. It includes hitting, kicking, punching, burning, tying up, or injuring or threatening with a weapon, such as a fist, knife, or gun.

*Sexual abuse* is any act of a sexual nature that hurts someone physically or emotionally, whether or not the person consents to the act. This type of abuse may be committed by a family member, spouse, friend, or stranger.

Rape is a violent form of sexual abuse. Child sexual abuse occurs when an adult uses a child for his own or another adult's sexual stimulation. Child sexual abuse may also be committed by someone who's under the age of 18 if he's either considerably older than the victim or he's in a position of power over the victim.

*Emotional abuse* ranges from indifference to verbal threats that erode the victim's self-esteem and security and cause fear or uncertainty. It includes excessive yelling, scolding, belittling, teasing, or criticizing. It can be as psychologically harmful as physical or sexual abuse and usually accompanies these forms of abuse.

*Neglect* is the failure to provide for a dependent person's basic needs, such as food, clothing, shel-

## Myths and truths about abuse

To combat the overwhelming incidence of abuse, you can help your patients replace common misconceptions about abuse with the facts.

**MYTH**
It won't happen to me.

**TRUTH**
All people are potential victims of abuse and violent crimes, but children, women, and elderly people are most vulnerable. Age, race, religion, socioeconomic class, and education don't protect a person from violence.

**MYTH**
A husband can't rape his wife. It's her duty to have sex with him.

**TRUTH**
This may have been legally true a century ago, but now wife battery and rape are illegal. A woman always has a right to say "no" to sex.

**MYTH**
Women who stay with abusive husbands must enjoy the abuse.

**TRUTH**
Leaving an abusive situation isn't that simple. An abused woman may fear that her abuser will come after her, or she may not be able to provide financially for herself or her children.

ter, hygiene, medical care, and supervision. With children, neglect also includes failing to provide the basic love and nurturing necessary for them to develop into productive members of society.

### Challenges in patient care
Nurses play a critical role in the detection and treatment of abuse because they're often the first ones to see a victim after abuse has occurred. And because most adult victims — and most nurses — are female, nurses are in a unique position to help these patients.

Caring for abused patients presents special challenges. You may find that your patient has some misconceptions about abuse, which you'll have to dispel before you can deliver effective care. (See *Myths and truths about abuse.*) You'll also discover that confirming abuse isn't always easy because some injuries that occur from abuse can also occur by accident.

What's more, patients often won't admit they're abused out of fear or shame. So you should expect some problem behaviors — passivity, depression, emotional instability, or even open hostility — when talking with the patient. Nevertheless, try to be understanding. Hospitalization or illness may be especially overwhelming to these patients whose coping mechanisms are already stressed to the limit, and who already feel vulnerable and dependent.

You'll also find that most patients won't discuss the abuse until you've developed a trusting relationship with them. Start building one by showing sensitivity and concern, giving them privacy, and trying not to react negatively or pass judgment. If the suspected abuser is present, you may have trouble staying calm, professional, and nonjudgmental around him. And yet you should, because helping the abuser will ultimately help the patient.

**MYTH**
People who abuse others are usually poor and have little education.

**TRUTH**
Abusers can come from any social class. In fact, most are well educated and come from upper-middle-class families.

**MYTH**
The media have blown the child sexual abuse problem out of proportion.

**TRUTH**
Sexual assault of children is widespread. An estimated 25% to 30% of women and 16% of men were sexually abused during childhood.

**MYTH**
Most rapes are committed by strangers.

**TRUTH**
Between 75% and 85% of victims know their attacker.

You'll also need to know certain legal aspects of abuse, including which cases must be reported to the police and what legal options are open to your patient. In rape cases, you must know what evidence is required and how to obtain it. In addition, you should be familiar with community resources and support services so that you can refer the patient and family to them. (See *Help for the abused and the abuser,* page 166.)

# Child abuse

Child abuse involves any type of action by adults that is physically or psychologically destructive to a child's well-being and normal growth and development. Child abuse occurs among all socioeconomic and ethnic groups and happens as often to boys as it does to girls — although girls are more likely to be the victims of sexual abuse. It often recurs in families. A child can be abused by anyone he comes into contact with — a teacher, family friend, baby-sitter, neighbor, or relative. So keep your eyes open to the possibility of abuse. Any questionable injury in a child should arouse your suspicion. Become familiar with child abuse laws and reporting practices and with your hospital and community resources.

**Assessment**
Child abuse is hard to pinpoint. The same injuries that result from abuse can also occur by accident. If you suspect child abuse, try to confirm it by evaluating the child's physical condition, behavior, and family situation. If you identify one factor that suggests abuse, always look for others to confirm your suspicions.

*Physical assessment.* Ask the parents to step out of the room so that

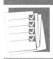

# Help for the abused and the abuser

Help can be just a phone call away for both the abused and the abuser. The national organizations listed below offer support and counseling, as do many community-based organizations. Give your patient the appropriate numbers from the list below. You can ask your hospital's social services department for help in finding local organizations.
☐ National Clearinghouse on Marital and Date Rape: (415) 524-1582
☐ National Coalition Against Sexual Assault: (202) 483-7165
☐ National Committee for the Prevention of Child Abuse: (312) 663-3520
☐ National Domestic Violence Hotline: (800) 333-SAFE
☐ Parents Anonymous: (800) 421-0353
☐ Parents United: (408) 453-7616

you and the doctor can provide emergency care, if needed. Once you've stabilized the child, perform a thorough physical examination. Keep in mind that the physical signs of child abuse differ according to the type of abuse.

*Physical abuse.* Inspect the child's skin over his entire body. Does he have cigarette burns, adult-sized bite marks, immersion burns, bald spots, lacerations or abrasions, welts and multiple bruises in various stages of healing, or genital injuries? Are the child's injuries symmetrical, indicating that they didn't occur naturally? Sites of abuse, in order of frequency, are the buttocks, hips, face, arms, back, and thighs.

Take special note of the pattern of multiple bruises. When children fall, bruising usually occurs on the

knees, shins, forehead, nose, or other bony prominences. Bruising on the buttocks, lower back, and lower thigh may be caused by paddling. Bruising on the earlobes suggests that they were pulled or pinched. Upper arm bruises can occur from being held tightly or grabbed forcefully. Bizarre markings result when a child is abused with such objects as a hot iron, a rope, or a belt buckle. Be sure to document the location, size, and approximate age of any bruises. (See *Estimating the age of a bruise.*) Also check the child's records to see if he has been treated in the past for similar injuries.

Next, assess the child for signs of neurologic damage. Blows to the head or violent shaking can injure the brain and spinal column. During infancy, this can cause mental retardation, blindness, or cerebral palsy. Subdural hematomas and other serious intracranial injuries in a child's first year are caused by physical abuse 95% of the time. If the child has a head injury, ask the parents about signs and symptoms of subdural hematoma, including headache, vomiting, hemiparesis, seizures, drowsiness, irritability, or personality changes.

*Sexual abuse.* In private, ask the child about any pain or itching in the genital area or difficulty walking or sitting. Inspect the perineum for genital lacerations, rectal tears, inflammation, vaginal discharge in girls (unusual at this age), or blood in stools. Because oral sex commonly occurs, inspect the child's mouth and throat for irritation and signs of venereal disease, such as herpetic ulcers. Also check for a hyperactive gag reflex and signs of vomiting, which may occur after a child has been forced to participate in oral sex.

Some children may show no visible signs of sexual abuse. But if you still suspect this problem, look for other clues, such as torn, stained, or bloody underclothes (in an emergency department patient) or, in girls, a history of urinary tract or yeast infections with no known medical cause. The doctor will order diagnostic tests to detect sexually transmitted diseases. Also look for behavioral clues, such as precocious sexual behavior or remarks.

*Emotional abuse.* Signs and symptoms of emotional abuse include speech disorders, delayed physical development, ulcers, asthma, severe allergies, and substance abuse. Evaluate the child for these problems through examination, observation, interviews with parents, and medical records, if available.

*Neglect.* Suspect neglect if the child is unusually dirty or smelly and inappropriately dressed for the weather. During your history, ask the child if he often feels hungry or if he's left alone without supervision for long periods of time.

Remember that young children may not have a correct concept of time, so determine the time frame by asking what show is on television when he gets home from school and what show is on when his parents come home.

During your physical examination, note signs that the child isn't receiving proper nutrition or hygiene. For example, are his teeth in poor condition? Is his abdomen distended? Does he show signs of vitamin deficiency, such as rickets? Does he have head lice?

**Behavioral assessment.** Assess the child's behavior while you're examining him and while he interacts

ASSESSMENT TIP

## Estimating the age of a bruise

Does your patient have multiple bruises? Use the chart below to estimate the age of the bruises and to help confirm that abuse has occurred.

| AGE OF BRUISE | COLOR AND APPEARANCE |
|---|---|
| 0 to 2 days | Red and puffy |
| 2 to 5 days | Blue to purple |
| 5 to 7 days | Green |
| 7 to 10 days | Yellow |
| 10 to 14 days | Yellow to brown (Skin clears in 2 to 4 weeks.) |

with other staff members and his parents. Note his facial expression and emotional responsiveness. Does he look apathetic, depressed, withdrawn, expressionless, or anxious? Does he pull away from his parents or cling to them? Does he seem guarded, as if he mistrusts others? Does he react inappropriately? (For example, does he say he's fine while he's crying?) Does he respond to others the same way as other children his age? Remember that "normal" behavior varies widely, so don't jump to conclusions.

Ask the parents about changes in the child's behavior. Has he had nightmares, enuresis, stomach aches, or increased crying spells? Does he startle easily? Does he want to avoid certain people or places? These may all be signs of child abuse.

Remember that the behavior of an abused child varies, depending on

## Detecting specific types of child abuse

If you think a child has been abused, but you're not sure exactly how, observe his behavior carefully. You'll commonly find specific patterns of behavior associated with each type of abuse.

### Physical abuse
The child who has suffered physical abuse may:
• complain of pain
• move as if he has been physically injured
• wear concealing clothing, even in hot weather
• avoid physical contact
• act either hostile and aggressive or timid and withdrawn
• try to hurt himself
• stay away from home as much as possible or run away from home.

### Sexual abuse
The sexually abused child may:
• sit or move gingerly
• display an obsession with his genitalia
• have few, if any, friends
• seem afraid of physical contact
• know much more about sex than other children his age

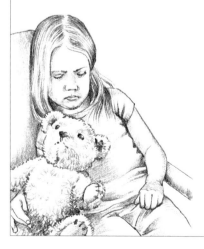

• appear introverted or depressed
• behave seductively
• have trouble falling asleep or other sleep problems, such as enuresis
• have recently lost or gained a great deal of weight
• suddenly start doing poorly in school
• fear being alone
• display self-destructive or suicidal behavior
• seem unwilling to take part in sports, take a shower, or perform any activity that calls for him to change his clothes
• seem unusually concerned about his siblings' safety
• try to avoid a particular person or persons.

### Emotional abuse
The child who has been emotionally abused may:
• rock, suck his thumb, or display another habit disorder
• fall behind in development
• behave in a disruptive or destructive manner
• have nightmares, enuresis, or other sleep problems
• abuse drugs or alcohol.

### Neglect
The neglected child may:
• be in the lowest third of a standard growth chart
• fall behind in development
• frequently miss school
• seem tired or fall asleep in class
• appear dirty, unkempt, or inappropriately dressed
• have impaired communication skills
• look undernourished and steal or beg for food from classmates
• have rashes, impetigo, scabies, or other skin problems
• have poor hand-eye coordination
• be accident-prone
• seldom smile or show emotion
• sleep poorly.

the type of abuse. (See *Detecting specific types of child abuse*.) To confirm your suspicions about the type of abuse, talk to the child privately and ask him direct questions, once you've gained his trust. Ask, "Has anyone hit you or hurt you? Has anyone touched you in private places? Can you tell me who?"

**Family assessment.** If you strongly suspect abuse, interview the parents and evaluate the home environment and family relationship for risk factors. (See *Risk factors for abuse in families*, this page, and *Characteristics of the abusive parent*, page 170.) Promote cooperation by reassuring the parents, offering support, and ensuring privacy. Then ask open-ended questions that require more than a one-word response and that give you a picture of the family situation and the child's usual behavior.

Ask for a detailed account of how the injury occurred, then observe the parents' response. Do they appear overly apologetic? Do they blame the child or siblings for the injury? Do they become angry or defensive? Do they seem unconcerned or overly concerned about the child? Do they say that they don't know where the injury came from? Does their explanation of what happened fail to match the child's injury or developmental stage? Did they delay seeking medical attention? Do they offer a partial "confession"? All of these responses point to child abuse.

If you think a child has been sexually abused, ask the parents about their normal routine, child care arrangements, and the child's behavior. For example, does the child spend a lot of time with a another caregiver? (If so, the parents may be unaware of the abuse.) Does he

CHECKLIST

## Risk factors for abuse in families

The more risk factors present in a family, the more likely it is that some type of abuse will occur. Risk factors include:
- ☐ a family history of abuse
- ☐ an unplanned pregnancy
- ☐ a difficult childbearing experience
- ☐ neonatal bonding problems
- ☐ alcohol or drug abuse in a family member
- ☐ financial problems
- ☐ housing problems
- ☐ health problems
- ☐ other marital problems
- ☐ psychological immaturity of the parents
- ☐ excessively strict discipline
- ☐ poor understanding of child growth and development.

routinely sleep with a parent or another adult? Has he ever shown precocious sexual behavior?

Be aware that in families where sexual abuse occurs, members are often abnormally absorbed in each other, and parent-child relationships are excessively close. Friendships outside the immediate family are discouraged, and physical and emotional boundaries are poorly established within the family. Oddly, if only one parent is abusive, he's commonly the more nurturing of the two.

Do you suspect emotional abuse? Families are emotionally abusive when they underestimate or overestimate a child's physical and emotional needs and place excessive demands on him. Then, when he can't meet those demands, they verbally abuse the child, creating in him a negative self-image. If you think this is the case with your pa-

## Characteristics of the abusive parent

An abusive parent isn't easy to spot. Although he probably won't display any obvious psychiatric problems, he may:
☐ have frequent bouts of depression
☐ demand too much from the child
☐ feel insecure and unloved himself and look toward the child to give him the support and comfort he wants
☐ believe that the child exists primarily to satisfy his needs
☐ consider the child's needs unimportant
☐ project his problems onto the child and then deal with his frustration with these problems by attacking the child
☐ have suffered abuse himself as a child.

tient, ask the parents how often they scold the child. How do they correct him when he hasn't met their expectations? Also observe the interaction between the child and the parents, and note how both parents react when the child doesn't perform up to their expectations.

Has the child obviously been neglected? Child neglect can result from ignorance, lack of education, or inadequate finances, or when the child isn't wanted or doesn't meet the parents' expectations. So be sure to assess the parents' educational level and financial status when you see signs of neglect in a child. Also carefully observe the interaction between the parents and the child.

### Intervention
Intervention begins during your first contact with the child and parents. Your goal is to protect the child's health and well-being and to provide as much consistency as possible in his life.

After your assessment, assist the doctor in treating any minor injuries. Then try to recognize your own feelings about child abuse. Although you can't help feeling angry at the abuser and sympathetic toward the child, try to avoid negative facial expressions or comments. The child might misinterpret your reaction as criticism and only feel more ashamed, and the parents might become even more defensive and refuse to cooperate.

*Treating the child.* Not every abused child has serious enough injuries to require hospitalization, but whenever possible, a child who may be the victim of abuse should be admitted for further treatment and evaluation. When abuse is strongly suspected, the doctor can hospitalize the child for up to 72 hours, even against the family's wishes.

When treating the child, first provide for his immediate needs, including safety, food, clothing, and hygiene. Victims of abuse or neglect are commonly deprived of these very basic needs. Next, provide positive feedback to help the child feel better about himself. He usually has low self-esteem and feels unworthy of love or attention. He may express negative feelings about himself. Your caring and encouragement will help alleviate some of his anxiety and allow you to build a trusting relationship.

Keep track of the child's visitors, and note how he reacts when he's around various people. Encourage him to talk about his feelings, but don't make judgmental comments. Give him drawing materials and other playthings, such as stuffed animals. Some children will alleviate their anxiety and act out their feelings of low self-esteem, fear, anger, and guilt through play.

Finally, make appropriate psychiatric and social service referrals so that the child will receive the support and follow-up care he needs to cope with his problems.

***Helping the family.*** If the parents are the abusers, they also need your help. This won't be easy, but try to show them some compassion and understanding, without justifying their abusive behavior. Being confrontational or accusatory will only frighten the child and his parents and put them on the defensive.

When the opportunity arises, talk to the parents about the child's good qualities and how much you like caring for him. Suggest some activities they might enjoy as a family, or demonstrate some simple games, then encourage them to join in with you and the child.

If appropriate, teach the parents about the normal growth and development of children, and discuss realistic expectations for various ages. Encourage any attempts by the parents to show appropriate love and affection for the child.

Also offer appropriate supportive therapy by making referrals to a social worker, family therapist, or marriage counselor.

***Legal interventions.*** Nurses working with children need to understand and obey the laws that concern the reporting of child abuse. Obviously, reporting child abuse is a delicate matter that requires careful and complete documentation. In all states, confirmed abuse must be reported to state authorities. In some states, suspected abuse also must be reported. The reporting procedure varies from state to state, so familiarize yourself with your state's law

and with your hospital's policy on handling child abuse.

Once abuse is reported, your state's child protective services agency will evaluate the situation further. The agency may require you to withhold the information from the parents so that they won't kidnap the child or pressure him to change his story before the investigation. Or the agency may require you to inform the parents that you've reported the abuse. If so, be sure the parents understand that the purpose of investigation is to help the family by providing information and support. Before acting, check the agency's policy manual for guidelines, and if you're still uncertain what to do, call the office for advice.

## Evaluation

Were your interventions successful? The answer to this question is yes if you and the child have developed a trusting relationship and he's beginning to trust others. If he's hospitalized long enough, you'll also begin to notice changes in his behavior — he'll be more relaxed, less depressed, and more willing to talk about the abuse.

Consider your interventions with the parents successful if they're learning new ways to cope with the stress of child rearing and if their words and actions show that they better understand their own and their child's needs. They also should be taking steps to resolve any drug and alcohol problems, which may have contributed to the child abuse.

If you learn during follow-up visits that the child is having school problems, sleeping problems (such as nightmares or enuresis), or personality problems, he may need long-term treatment and further psychiatric evaluation.

# Spouse abuse

An estimated 11% to 34% of people in the United States are abused by their spouses or sexual partners. Apparently, many cases go unreported because the victim is ashamed or fears reprisal. Although occasionally the man is the abused partner, and in some relationships both partners are abusive, most victims are women, who are physically weaker than men and often socially and economically dependent on them.

A national crime survey taken from 1978 to 1982 estimated that in a 12-month period, 2.1 million women were victims at least once of rape, robbery, or assault by their partners. One-third of these women were victimized again within 6 months. Studies show that women may be at increased risk for physical abuse during pregnancy. In selected populations, as many as 63% of women were physically abused during pregnancy. Studies also reveal that these women are four times more likely to deliver low-birth-weight infants.

Spouse abuse is devastating to the whole family and is commonly grounds for divorce. Children from such families usually have behavioral problems, may be abused themselves, or may grow up to be abusers. Many abused women eventually develop psychiatric problems.

## Assessment

Typically, spouse abuse is easier to diagnose than child abuse. That's because adults simply don't hurt themselves accidentally as much as children do. But you still need to assess patients carefully. Confirm your suspicions through a thorough physical examination, a family assessment, and an assessment of the patient's behavior.

*Physical assessment.* Your first priority — before attempting to determine whether the patient has in fact been abused — is to assess and treat her physical injuries. Be sure to conduct the examination in private, away from the patient's partner. As you're helping her undress, check her clothes for bloodstains or tears. Typical injuries include multiple bruises and lacerations (in various stages of healing) on the face, neck, breasts, abdomen, back, and genitalia; fractured limbs; dislocated joints; internal injuries; and cigarette burns, rope burns, or other unusual or oddly shaped injuries. Document the location and size of each injury carefully.

In addition, patients may have chronic problems or vague complaints, such as headaches, abdominal pain, sexual dysfunction, recurrent vaginal infections, joint pains, muscle aches, or sleep and eating disorders.

During your examination, also note (or ask) whether the patient is pregnant because pregnant women are at increased risk for physical abuse. And check the patient's records to see if she's ever been admitted before with suspicious injuries.

*Family assessment.* Once the physical injuries are cared for, try to determine their cause. Interview the patient in private, but don't be surprised if her partner tries to interrupt the interview. Approach the patient gently, with acceptance and understanding, so that she'll trust you enough to confide her problems. Try to piece together the couple's situation by asking the patient questions about her current injury and any past injuries. How did she get these injuries? Did her partner cause them? Has he ever hurt her before or hurt others? Has he ever humiliated her? Taken her money? Threatened her or her family? Has she tried to get help? If so, what was the outcome? Is she afraid to return home? What other options does she have?

Also be alert for vague explanations or inconsistencies in the patient's description of how the injury occurred. For example, if her arm is broken, she might say that her partner just shoved her slightly. Or the patient's description of how the injury occurred might contradict other family members' stories. For instance, a pregnant woman might claim that she tripped and fell down the stairs, bruising her abdomen, whereas her sister might report that the woman was arguing with her intoxicated boyfriend when she was hurt.

If such inconsistencies occur, delve deeper into the woman's home situation and relationship with her partner. Is she under a lot of stress at home? Does she often have disagreements with her partner? How do they usually resolve these situations? If they fight, do the fights escalate from yelling to physical contact? Do either of them abuse alcohol or drugs? (See *Characteristics of the abusive man,* page 174.) Encourage the patient to reveal important information, and let her know you're on her side by trying not to overreact or be judgmental during questioning. For example, you might use this wording: "Your injuries could be caused by someone hitting you. Has anyone done this?"

***Behavioral assessment.*** Be aware that many women are too ashamed or frightened to admit that they're abused. So observe the patient's behavior closely during your examination and interview, checking for clues to abuse. For example, is she withdrawn, passive, or indifferent during your assessment? Does she laugh inappropriately, avoid eye contact, sigh frequently, cry or become tearful, use anxious body language, play down her problem, become defensive, or start talking about someone she knows who has been abused?

Also assess the patient for symptoms of posttraumatic stress disorder (PTSD), which is associated with prolonged abuse. Suspect PTSD if the patient admits to having intrusive and fearful thoughts and shows a lack of responsiveness, social withdrawal, diminished interest in normal activities, irritability, and an increased startle response.

Finally, remember that suicide attempts are common in victims of spouse abuse. So ask the patient if she has ever attempted suicide or thought about harming herself.

### Intervention
Once the patient has been identified as an abuse victim, concentrate on helping her cope with her situation. For instance, help her decide where to go and what to do next. Tell her what kind of help is available in the community and make her aware of legal actions she can take. If she's determined to return to the abusive partner, help her devise a plan of action to keep her and her children safe.

***Discussing options with the patient.*** Once abuse has been determined, help the patient repair her life. You can't tell her what to do, even though you'd probably like to. But you can help her explore her op-

## Characteristics of the abusive man

Men who abuse their partners commonly share several characteristics. An abusive man may:
□ have a successful career
□ act sensitive, charming, affectionate, or seductive toward his partner in public but jealous, possessive, impulsive, impatient, angry, or intimidating toward her in private
□ fail to recognize his behavior as inappropriate
□ blame his partner for everything that goes wrong in his life
□ abuse drugs or alcohol
□ claim that women have betrayed him
□ feel threatened and demeaned by women
□ describe his father as a weak man
□ describe his mother as domineering
□ have witnessed or experienced abuse while growing up.

tions. For example, she can get out of the abusive relationship and live with a relative until she gets back on her feet. Or she can return home as long as her partner agrees to go with her for counseling. Or she can simply go back and try to avoid being abused again. Talking about the nature, pattern, and frequency of abuse in her life and how she copes will help her face her problem and possibly avoid future abusive relationships.

*Leaving the relationship.* The patient may feel that she has nowhere to go and no one to turn to. Help her feel less isolated by discussing possible support systems — for example, her family, the clergy, community support groups, counselors, or shelters for battered women. She may also be able to get the abuser to leave the house. Hospital staff members can help her accomplish this, but only with the partner's co-operation. If he won't agree to leave or threatens to hurt her, her children, or other family members, the patient should leave home instead.

If this happens, help her find a suitable place to stay. If she can't stay with a relative or friend, help her find temporary housing through a social service agency. If all else fails, refer the patient to a shelter for battered women. Ask your hospital social service department for a list of shelters in your area, or contact the National Domestic Violence Hotline at 1-800-333-SAFE. Staying in a shelter is very disruptive to families, so the patient will need support during this time.

*Staying in the relationship.* If the patient wants to return to her abusive partner, try to avoid being judgmental. Ask her why she wants to go back after such a traumatic incident and if she thinks that she'll be safe. Let her know you're concerned for her safety. Make sure that she has a place to go when the threat of abuse is imminent. Before she leaves the hospital, help her prepare a plan for avoiding further abuse or for seeking shelter after it occurs. (See *Planning ahead to escape abuse.*)

In all cases, refer the patient to an outpatient counselor, especially if she seems suicidal or shows signs of PTSD. Group therapy may be especially helpful because it provides a support group for the patient. Group therapy also helps her identify her strengths, learn the dynamics of abuse, and find new ways to cope. If the abusive partner requests counseling, couple therapy might be recommended — but usually not until

## Planning ahead to escape abuse

If your patient decides to return to her abusive partner after treatment, you can't stop her—even though you'd like to. But you can help her develop a plan of action to use when abuse seems imminent or after it has occurred. Planning ahead will increase her chances of escaping to a safe place, with her children if she has any. Here are some steps she can take.

☐ *Choose a method of transportation.* If the patient has a car, help her decide on a safe place to hide an extra set of keys. (Make sure she chooses a place her abuser won't find.) If she doesn't have a car, she can hide fare money and a bus schedule or the phone number for a cab company.

☐ *Choose possible destinations.* Have her list the names and phone numbers of people she can go to in an emergency. If she's unsure whether she can stay with someone, she can call from the hospital to double-check.

Also, help her list the addresses and phone numbers of shelters in her area. She can hide the lists with her cab fare, bus schedule, or car keys.

☐ *Pack a few belongings.* If possible, she should keep a few belongings at one of the "safe" homes on her list. Or, if she has a car, she can keep a change of clothes and a few personal items in the trunk, in case she needs to make a quick escape.

☐ *Save some money.* Encourage the patient to start saving small amounts of money, if possible. She can keep the money in her hiding place.

☐ *Gather important papers.* Help her make a list of important papers she'll need if she leaves home. She can hide these papers along with the items mentioned above.

☐ *Find someone who will call the police.* Suggest that she confide in a neighbor, if possible, who can call the police if she hears sounds of violence.

both partners have received individual therapy for several months.

***Legal interventions.*** Nurses caring for victims of spouse abuse must be familiar with the reporting requirements and procedures for initiating legal action. Spouse abuse may constitute assault and battery. Although only the patient can bring charges in these cases, you can provide support. However, if the patient is otherwise physically and mentally fit, you're usually under no legal obligation to notify your state's protective services agency.

Be sure to inform the patient of her legal rights and reassure her that assistance is available. Explain that she can obtain a temporary re-

straining order from the local courthouse, written to include specific restrictions to meet her needs. She also can contact the police after abuse has occurred and file a report, even if she doesn't want to file criminal charges against her partner at the time. This documentation can be used as evidence for future legal actions, if necessary.

### Evaluation

Most abuse victims will eventually leave their partners or try to stop or at least reduce the abuse. But because most of them cling to the hope that their partners will reform, they usually first undergo multiple separations and reunions. So don't try to base the success of your nursing interventions solely on the fact that the couple has separated. Instead, consider your work successful if the abused partner recognizes that she has a problem, understands the extent of the problem and its impact on her physical and emotional health as well as its impact on her children, and knows what options are available to her.

Evaluate the effectiveness of your interventions by asking yourself these questions:
• Is the patient safer now?
• Does she understand how community resources can help, and does she have a list of places to contact?
• Have the two of you developed an alternative plan should the abuse recur?

# Elder abuse

Many elderly people become dependent on others because of poor health or financial problems. This makes them especially vulnerable to abuse and, most commonly, chronic passive neglect. Elders at greatest risk are frail, white, Protestant women over age 75 who have multiple physical, mental, and emotional problems; are disoriented; and are dependent on others for nutrition, safety, and toileting. In most cases, the abuser is a close relative, such as a spouse or an adult child.

What causes elder abuse? One common theory is that violence is a learned pattern in some families and that people who were abused as children may later abuse their elderly parents in revenge. According to another theory, the relative has so much external stress (for example, from his job or children) that he can't care for the elderly person

properly and ends up abusing or neglecting her.

## Assessment

Elder abuse can be difficult to confirm because many victims won't admit they're abused for fear of losing their only means of support. In addition, some patients are too mentally impaired to provide a history of the abuse. So when examining an elderly patient, always be alert to the possibility of passive neglect and mistreatment.

Assess the patient's physical, mental, and emotional health and family situation. When possible, perform your examination without another family member present so that the patient can speak freely. Also, try to establish a trusting relationship with the patient.

*Physical assessment.* If the patient has any acute injuries, treat them first. Then perform a routine physical examination, maintaining privacy at all times. Inspect the skin for bruises or lacerations, looking for any unusual patterns. Remember that elderly skin is fragile, so injuries can sometimes occur with normal activity.

However, multiple bruises or lacerations in various stages of healing can signify abuse, especially if they appear on the upper arms, back, buttocks, and thighs. Contractures, rope burns, or bruising in the corners of the mouth can signal that the patient has been restrained for a long time.

Pressure ulcers in advanced stages, dehydration, and malnourishment can also be signs of abuse or neglect. So weigh the patient and carefully assess skin turgor. Document all your findings, noting the exact locations and sizes of injuries as well as the approximate age of any bruises. Precise documentation is essential from a medical and legal standpoint.

**Mental and emotional assessment.** Start by evaluating the patient's mental status, using the Goldfarb 10-point scale. Next, establish the patient's level of independence by having her describe an average day. Can she prepare her own meals, shop for groceries, pay her bills, bathe herself, and perform other self-care activities?

If she says that she needs help, ask who usually provides it. Then watch for any verbal or nonverbal clues that might signal abuse or neglect when she mentions the helpers. If a facial expression or gesture concerns you, ask the patient to tell you what she's thinking. For example, you might say, "I noticed that you frowned and looked at the floor when you mentioned your daughter. Has she done anything to upset you lately?"

If the patient admits to feeling hopeless or depressed, ask her what has happened recently to make her feel this way and what would make her feel better. Also inquire if she has felt neglected or mistreated recently or in the past. If she says yes, ask her to be more specific: Has she ever been physically harmed or deprived of care and necessities? Can she describe these episodes?

Such questions can reveal a pattern of abuse and allow the patient to report a previous incident. They can also distance her from the current situation and relieve her discomfort about reporting a close relative. Asking about the past also taps the patient's long-term memory, which may be more intact than her short-term memory. Use direct quotes from the patient when documenting your findings.

**Family assessment.** After performing a physical assessment and evaluating the patient's mental and emotional status, talk to family members. Ask what type of care the patient requires and if the family is having any trouble providing it.

Assess the family for signs of stress, frustration, or anger toward the patient, once again looking for verbal and nonverbal clues that might suggest abuse or neglect. For example, are they blaming the patient for her physical problems, being overly defensive, or showing little concern for her well-being? Do they seem overly tense, irritable, or resentful? Do they make statements such as "I'm sick of having to clean up after her in the bathroom"?

If you noticed signs of abuse or neglect during the physical examination, ask the family if they know how these problems occurred. If any problems are in advanced stages, such as malnourishment or pressure ulcers, ask why they didn't seek medical attention sooner.

Also assess the financial situation of the patient and family. Does the patient live alone or with the family? Does the patient's social security check go into a personal account, or does a family member deposit it into his own account? Does the patient have any control over her finances? Is the person caring for the patient controlling the patient's finances?

If the patient requires hospitalization, take this opportunity to assess the extent of family support. How often do family members visit? How do they interact with the patient? Watch for any unusual family interactions. Also, start a conversation about the patient's care to see how the family reacts. You might gather valuable information to help you identify the potential for abuse.

## Intervention

When the assessment is finished, help the doctor treat any minor injuries. Then work toward the goal of providing for the patient's safety by encouraging open communication between the patient and family. Urge the patient to discuss her feelings with her family—then note how they interact. Also, offer the family emotional support, empathy, and concrete suggestions for relieving stress.

***Increasing patient independence.*** With the family present, review any prescribed medications to be sure the patient is taking them correctly. If she has a complicated medication regimen, suggest that she use a multidose dispenser that has the day and time for each dose marked on the container. Make sure she or another family member knows how to fill and use the dispenser.

Be alert for possible drug interactions that could cause physical or emotional problems. If the patient has any physical problems that could cause cognitive impairment or emotional instability, refer her for appropriate treatment. Also, teach the family about the normal aging process so that they know what to expect.

These steps may increase the patient's independence and relieve family stress, lessening the risk of further abuse or neglect. Sometimes, elderly patients are capable of doing more than the family realizes. In these cases, ask an occupational therapist to assess the patient's abilities and weaknesses so that he can help her maximize her strengths.

***Reducing family stress.*** Obtain a social history from the family to determine their stress level. If one person is providing most of the patient's care, encourage him to involve other family members or close friends so that he won't feel so overwhelmed. Sharing the responsibility makes other family members aware of the patient's care requirements, decreasing family tensions.

Remember that interpersonal conflicts often underlie abuse. How the family reacts and adapts to the presence of a dependent older relative varies, depending on the roles of the patient and the abuser; the ages, personalities, and health of other family members; the family's living conditions; and financial concerns such as college expenses.

***Finding outside help.*** In many cases, elder abuse could be prevented if the families realized that community resources are available to help. So make referrals as needed to local home health care agencies, visiting nurse or homemaker services, day care programs, and respite care facilities. These services are geared to elderly patients who function at varying levels and can provide a social outlet to minimize their isolation. They can also reduce family tensions by providing respite care.

If the patient was hospitalized, home health care agencies and visiting nurse associations can provide follow-up care. Welfare or family service agencies can provide additional support and even offer financial assistance. Other community resources, such as support groups for families of patients with Alzheimer's disease, give family members a chance to share information and vent their frustrations.

***Seeking psychiatric help.*** If the patient shows signs of depression, such as decreased appetite, low energy level, or apathy, or if she talks about committing suicide, ask for a psychiatric consultation. Also keep in mind that confusion, combativeness, and restlessness can be symptoms of depression but are often mistaken for dementia.

A psychiatrist or psychiatric clinical nurse specialist can also help the family understand and cope with disorders such as Alzheimer's disease. For example, family members may think that the patient is acting childish just to get attention. But once they realize that she can't help this behavior, they'll be able to adjust better, and the potential for abuse should decrease.

***Ensuring patient safety.*** Once abuse is suspected or confirmed, the patient's safety is your priority. If you or anyone on the health care team believes that the patient is at risk for serious injury, recommend that she be separated from the abuser.

Consider all alternative placements, including relatives, friends, a shelter (unless the patient needs treatment for a medical problem), or a nursing home, even if the arrangement is only temporary. If the patient is competent, explain the options available, and ask her if she knows of any other possibilities.

Support her in whatever decision she makes. You can also call your state's adult protective services agency, which will contact the family and further assess the situation.

Failing to report abuse can lead to criminal or civil penalties, especially if the patient is in a boarding or nursing home. So become familiar with state laws and hospital protocol for reporting abuse, and thoroughly document evidence of abuse.

### Evaluation
Have your interventions been a success? Although you'll be able to assess the effectiveness of your physical care, you'll have to wait for the home health or visiting nurse's evaluation of your other interventions and referrals. Continued follow-up care and support are essential. If family members realize that they need help to cope, are receptive to referrals, and take steps to learn how to deal with the situation, your efforts have succeeded.

# Rape

Rape is a violent act of sexual aggression intended to humiliate and control another person. Victims range from the very young to the elderly and include both men and women. However, women are the victims in about 93% of documented cases. Unfortunately, no one knows the real number of rapes committed because anxiety, fear, embarrassment, and depression discourage many victims from reporting the crime or even seeking medical help. People who do seek treatment have special physical, emotional, and legal needs, which you must be aware of in order to provide quality care.

### Assessment
First and foremost, provide privacy for the rape victim. She's already traumatized, so keep the number of health care workers present to a minimum to help her feel less embarrassed and intimidated. She'll probably be extremely upset, agitated, and frightened, so offer constant emotional support during your assessment.

If the patient is physically injured, provide emergency care, but save more extensive treatment for later so that you don't destroy evi-

## Phases of rape-trauma syndrome

Most rape victims begin to experience rape-trauma syndrome about 24 hours after the attack. This syndrome usually occurs in three phases, although a patient won't necessarily experience them in sequence. These phases are characterized by the signs and symptoms listed below.

| PHASE | SIGNS AND SYMPTOMS |
|-------|--------------------|
| Acute | Anger, apprehension, denial, disbelief, fear, shock, vengefulness, and feelings of degradation, guilt, humiliation, and powerlessness. Victim may seek medical help or keep the rape a secret. |
| Outward adjustment | Appears calm. Denies real feelings but may try to take control by getting new door locks or buying a gun. May refuse emotional support and counseling. |
| Reorganization | Suffers from anxiety, phobias, sexual problems, and sleep problems. Wants to discuss feelings and work them out. May go for counseling and seek support from others or may continue to suffer silently. |

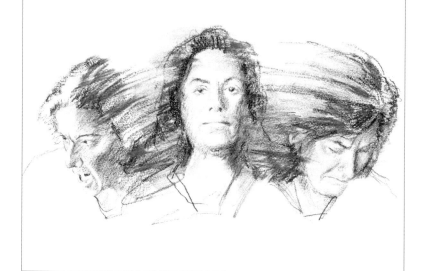

dence. If she's alone, ask if you can contact a family member or friend for additional support, but don't be surprised if she refuses out of shame and embarrassment. Explain that, by law, you must contact the police so that they can file a report, but that she can decide later whether or not to press charges.

Also call your local victim assistance agency and ask if they can send a rape counselor to stay with the patient throughout the examination and police report procedures. Once the patient is physically stable, perform a thorough assessment, following your state's laws for collecting evidence and your hospital's protocol for caring for a rape victim.

**Behavioral, emotional, and cognitive assessment.** First, assess the patient's ability to respond to questions about the rape. She may be too agitated, distraught, or confused to answer questions or even follow simple directions. Or she may be afraid to talk because the rapist has threatened to hurt her or her family if the police are notified. If the patient delayed coming to the hospital, also consider the possibility that she's experiencing rape-trauma syndrome. (See *Phases of rape-trauma syndrome.*)

If the patient is able, ask her to describe the rape, then record it in her own words. Seeing you write down her description might intensify her feelings of shame, so ensure complete privacy, and explain that the information will help the doctor determine the extent of her injuries and help you and the doctor plan her care. Next, obtain a sexual history. Ask the patient if she's sexually active, what form of birth control she uses, when she last had intercourse before the rape, and the date of her last menstrual period.

**Physical assessment.** Before beginning, explain the purpose of the rape examination, and have the patient sign a consent form. Help her change into a hospital gown, being careful how you handle her clothing, especially her undergarments. Circle any suspected blood or semen stains with a laundry marker. Fold each piece of clothing individually and place it in a brown paper bag to be

## Assessing the male rape victim

Men who've been raped also feel shame, fear, guilt, and embarrassment. So they need the same gentle consideration as female victims and the same prophylactic treatment for sexually transmitted diseases. Don't add to the patient's humiliation by implying that he's less masculine because of the rape or that a man can't be raped.

When assessing the patient, watch for these problems:
• bleeding from rectal tears.
• multiple internal or external injuries. Considerable violence usually accompanies male rape because both people are commonly of comparable strength. The victim may also have been gang raped.
• signs of drug or alcohol intoxication. The victim may have been drugged or encouraged to drink excessively before the attack.

given to the authorities. Don't use airtight plastic bags—they stimulate bacterial action that may alter the evidence.

Perform a head-to-toe assessment of the patient's skin, looking for cuts and bruises. Document the size, location, and age of any injuries and, if possible, photograph them. Injuries commonly associated with rape are cuts and bruises on the face, arms, breasts, thighs, and lower back. If a weapon was used, the patient's injuries will be more severe and may include puncture wounds, gunshot wounds, concussions, or internal injuries. Male rape victims commonly have more serious injuries than females. (See *Assessing the male rape victim.*)

Now you're ready to start the

### Easing the rape victim's distress

To ease a rape victim's distress, look for little ways to make her more comfortable during the physical examination and specimen collection. For example:
☐ Include the patient in your conversation with the doctor. Call her by name as you're talking to the doctor; don't refer to her indirectly, as if she's not there. Don't discuss unrelated topics with the doctor — this shows a lack of concern for the patient.
☐ Keep her body and legs covered as much as possible. Expose only those areas being examined.
☐ Warm the speculum and other examining instruments to room temperature.
☐ Stay with the patient after the examination to help her dress and to reassure her. Keep in mind that the examination itself could cause her to have a flashback of her assault.

rape examination. Explain each step as you go along, offering constant emotional support and giving positive feedback as the patient follows each step, to increase her sense of control. Be sure she understands that physical evidence must be obtained now — otherwise, prosecution is impossible. But tell her that she can decide later whether or not to press charges. (See *Easing the rape victim's distress*.)

Collect scrapings from underneath the patient's fingernails so that they can be examined for blood or skin fragments. Put the specimens in capped laboratory tubes, and label each appropriately. Comb the patient's pubic hair to collect foreign specimens — or let her do this herself. Let the hair fall onto a sheet of

paper and then place it in a labeled plastic bag. You also may need to take several strands of the patient's head hair to compare with other hair specimens found during the investigation.

Help the patient into the lithotomy position, and explain that the doctor will now perform a pelvic examination to collect semen specimens from the vagina, rectum, or urethra. Ask if she has ever had a pelvic examination and, if not, explain the procedure. The doctor also may take specimens from the patient's pharynx, if necessary. Explain that all the specimens will be cultured for gonorrhea.

Hold the patient's hand during the examination, and talk to her soothingly. Encourage her to let you and the doctor know if she feels any fear or discomfort or if she has any questions.

Remember to use only plain water or normal saline solution as a lubricant on the speculum because other lubricants may destroy evidence. Semen specimens dry out quickly, so deliver the specimens to the laboratory immediately; then wait for the results while the technician records the number of sperm per high-power field. (For permanent smears, the doctor will order a Papanicolaou test, a methylene blue test, or a gram stain.)

If the patient didn't report the rape right away, the doctor will assess her for venereal disease and pregnancy during the pelvic examination. However, he won't be able to do a rape examination because evidence will have been destroyed.

### Intervention

Once your assessment is completed and all specimens are obtained, assist the doctor in cleaning and treating any minor injuries. Continue to encourage the patient to express her feelings, which may help her regain a sense of control. Expect her to feel shame, guilt, powerlessness, anger, and fear, and to say such things as "I feel so dirty" or "I'll never be clean again" or "I want to kill him." Listen and offer support.

***Medications and diagnostic tests.*** At this point, the doctor may decide to administer medications to prevent tetanus or infection in open or contaminated wounds. He may also order medications to treat sexually transmitted diseases (STDs). You'll need to help him explain the purpose of these medications and then help him administer them to the patient. You'll also need to draw blood to test for STDs.

Also, warn the patient about the risk of pregnancy. If she chooses, the doctor will order diethylstilbestrol (DES), a postcoital contraceptive, to prevent pregnancy. Be sure to explain the risks of this drug and obtain a signed consent before administering the first dose. If your hospital doesn't offer pregnancy prophylaxis, refer the patient to another hospital. But don't pressure her — she may be too upset to make an informed decision, or she may be torn because of religious or cultural beliefs. Instead, reassure her that she has time to make the decision, and then explain her options: She can start taking DES within 72 hours after the rape (preferably within 24 hours), or she can wait and see if she's pregnant and then have an abortion if she chooses. Or she can have the child if she's pregnant. If she chooses to go through with the pregnancy, refer her to a counselor who can help her deal with any feelings of anger or revictimization that may evolve as the pregnancy progresses.

Explain to the patient that some tests may need to be repeated in 2 weeks and again in 6 weeks because not all STDs can be identified immediately after being transmitted. Warn her, too, of the danger of contracting acquired immunodeficiency syndrome (AIDS). Inform her that AIDS testing isn't accurate until at least 6 weeks after a potential infection, so she'll have to wait to be tested.

If she has a positive result from an STD test, you'll need to educate her about the disease and discuss further treatment options. If she tests positive for the human immunodeficiency virus, she'll need extensive education and counseling. Make sure you get the patient's forwarding address if she's moving or leaving town temporarily so that the hospital can mail her test results to her.

***Future safety.*** For a rape victim, the nightmare doesn't end when she leaves the hospital. She still has to deal with the fear of future attacks. Taking a course in self-defense or improving security at home will help her regain a sense of control over her life. So give her information on community programs or support groups, and suggest some simple changes she can make, such as putting deadbolt locks on her doors.

If the patient was raped by a family member, a friend, or an acquaintance, she probably won't feel safe upon first returning home. If she doesn't have a friend or relative to stay with temporarily, ask your hospital's social services department to help her find a safe place to live. If the patient decides to return home, help her devise a plan of action if rape seems imminent or occurs again.

**Legal interventions.** Ask the rape
counselor or another qualified person to explain the patient's legal
rights. Be sure the patient realizes
that she'll have to appear in court if
she decides to press charges. Advise
her to write down the details of the
rape while they're still fresh in her
mind, to help her during her testi-
mony.

**Emotional support.** Encourage the
patient to seek professional counseling to help her deal with her fear,
anxiety, and anger so that she can
try to regain her feelings of self-
worth and control and get on with
her life. Emphasize that rape isn't
an experience she can just "get
over." If the patient is married or in
a serious relationship, advise couple
counseling. Family counseling may
also help, depending on the reaction
of the patient's loved ones.

### Evaluation
Determining the success of your interventions will be difficult because
the victim will need time and counseling to deal with the rape. During
follow-up visits, a counselor will try
to determine whether the patient
thinks about the rape less often and
whether talking about it is less painful or frightening. He'll also find out
if the patient has been able to resume her normal life-style without
undue fears.

If the patient isn't making progress, the counselor may need to reevaluate her support systems and
consider the possibility of PTSD. If
she's talking about suicide, engaging in self-destructive behavior,
feeling anxious or depressed, afraid
to form new friendships, or shun-

ning old friends, the counselor may
make the appropriate referrals to a
psychiatrist or a psychiatric clinical
nurse specialist.

### Suggested readings
Bullock, L., et al. "Breaking the Cycle of
Abuse: How Nurses Can Intervene,"
*Journal of Psychosocial Nursing*
27(8):11-13, August 1989.
Campbell, J., and Sheridan, D. "Emer-
gency Nursing Interventions with Bat-
tered Women," *Journal of Emergency
Nursing* 15(1):12-17, January-February
1989.
Chez, R. "Woman Battering," *American
Journal of Obstetrics and Gynecology*
158(1):1-4, January 1988.
Danis, D., et al. "Battered Women Hand-
out and Referral Card," *Journal of
Emergency Nursing* 15(1):49-51, Janu-
ary-February 1989.
*Diagnostic and Statistical Manual of
Mental Disorders,* 3rd ed., revised.
Washington, D.C.: American Psychiat-
ric Association, 1987.
Dickstein, L.J., and Nadelson, C.C. *Fam-
ily Violence: Emerging Issues of a Na-
tional Crisis.* Washington, D.C.:
American Psychiatric Press, 1990.
Fulmer, T. "Elder Abuse," in *Abuse and
Victimization Across the Life Span.* Ed-
ited by Straus, M.D. Baltimore: Johns
Hopkins University Press, 1988.
Hartman, D. "Battered Women: The
Fight You Can Help Them Win,"
*NursingLife* 7(5):37-39, September-
October 1987.
Helfer, R.E., and Kemp, R.S. *The Bat-
tered Child,* 4th ed. Chicago: Univer-
sity of Chicago Press, 1987.
Johnson, C.F. "Child Abuse and the Child
Psychiatrist," in *Psychiatric Disorders
in Children and Adolescents.* Edited by
Garfinkel, B. Philadelphia: W.B. Saun-
ders Co., 1990.

# 11

# SUBSTANCE ABUSE

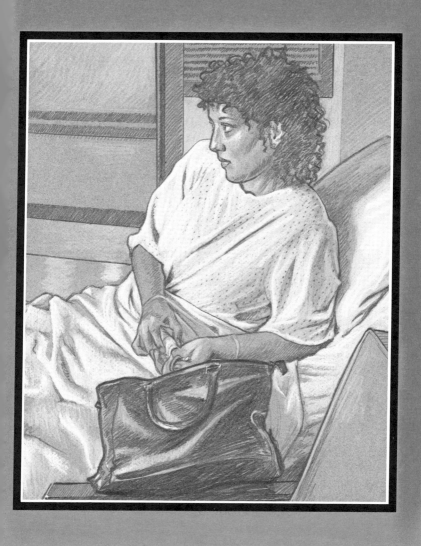

Excessive use of alcohol or other drugs, substance abuse is a public health concern that disrupts family and social relationships and creates hazards in the workplace. One of the major causes of work-related accidents, turnover, absenteeism, waste, and health care expenses, substance abuse is not limited to any specific socioeconomic, cultural, or age group. Substance abuse pervades our society, and you can expect to encounter it often, even if you don't specialize in psychiatric nursing.

This chapter helps you understand and recognize substance abuse so that you can intervene appropriately. First, you'll find a discussion of characteristics common to substance abusers and a discussion of the causes of substance abuse. The chapter then describes the differences between acute intoxication and chronic abuse to help you assess your patient accurately. Finally, the chapter outlines the various options available for treating the effects of acute intoxication and rehabilitating the chronic substance abuser.

# Understanding substance abuse

The *Diagnostic and Statistical Manual of Mental Disorders,* 3rd edition (revised), defines substance abuse as a maladaptive pattern of using psychoactive substances. The diagnosis is confirmed when a person continues to use the substance despite knowing about the possible hazards. When a person becomes addicted to the abused substance, physical or psychological dependence results. (See *Criteria for diagnosing psychoactive substance dependence.*)

Commonly abused substances include alcohol; inhalants, such as glue and gasoline; steroids; nicotine; prescription medications, such as antianxiety agents and narcotics; and street drugs, such as cocaine, phencyclidine (PCP), amphetamines and related stimulants, marijuana, and hallucinogens. All of these drugs, except for hallucinogens, can be addictive.

## Characteristics of substance abusers

Although any patient may have underlying substance dependence, the likelihood increases with certain medical conditions. Examples of such conditions include accidental injury, malnutrition, human immunodeficiency virus (HIV) infection, elective and emergency surgery, a newly diagnosed disease, and pregnancy. Once abuse has begun, a substance abuser also has a higher risk of certain health problems, such as hypertension and deterioration of brain and liver cells.

Many substance abusers share certain key personality traits. Although outwardly dominant and critical of others, a typical substance abuser is inwardly passive and full of self-doubt. His psychosocial development is arrested at an early stage. The substance abuser may act promiscuously, dress inappropriately, have trouble forming intimate relationships, and have problems with sexual identification.

A typical substance abuser relies on defense mechanisms, such as escapism, denial, and rationalization, to justify his behavior. Because he's prone to increased anxiety, depression, and mood swings, his relationships with others may become

# Criteria for diagnosing psychoactive substance dependence

According to the *Diagnostic and Statistical Manual of Mental Disorders,* 3rd edition (revised), a patient with psychoactive substance dependence exhibits at least three of the following:
• a need to take larger amounts of the substance over a longer period than the patient intended
• a persistent desire to stop or limit the use of the substance, or one or more unsuccessful attempts to end dependence
• a tendency to spend a great deal of time getting the substance, taking it, or recovering from its effects
• frequent intoxication or withdrawal symptoms when the patient is expected to fulfill major role obligations at work, school, or home
• a tendency to curtail or abandon important social, occupational, or recreational activities because of substance use

• continued abuse of the substance despite the knowledge that it causes or exacerbates a persistent or recurrent social, psychological, or physical problem
• a need to increase the amount of the substance taken by at least 50% to achieve the desired effect, or a markedly diminished effect when the same amount of the substance is used
• characteristic withdrawal symptoms (these vary depending on the substance abused)
• the need to take the substance to relieve or avoid withdrawal symptoms.

Some of these symptoms should have persisted for at least 1 month or have occurred repeatedly over a longer period of time. Also, the last two symptoms listed above may not apply to a patient who abuses cannabis (marijuana), hallucinogens, or phencyclidine (PCP).

impaired, causing tension, embarrassment, and family disruption. Poor work performance, financial difficulties, and criminal lawsuits may also stem from substance abuse.

Additional characteristics depend on whether the patient is abusing alcohol or other drugs.

***Alcohol abuse.*** A patient who abuses alcohol experiences irregular depression of the central nervous system (CNS). At lower concentrations, alcohol results in a release of inhibitions, feelings of relaxation, diminished tension and anxiety, and impaired judgment. Increasing levels cause impaired motor function, slurred speech, and staggered gait.

Alcoholism defies easy definition. The primary criterion for diagnosis is drinking behavior that interferes with a person's ability to carry out his usual daily activities or that adversely affects his interpersonal relationships. Excessive alcohol use can result in both physical and psychological dependence. Physical dependence occurs when the patient develops a biological need for alcohol; if it's not supplied, he suffers physical withdrawal symptoms. Psychological dependence occurs when the patient craves the effects of alcohol.

***Drug abuse.*** This term refers to the use of any mind-altering substance other than alcohol, except as prescribed by a doctor. Drug addiction may involve physical dependence, psychological dependence, or both. The combination of these two factors forms a powerful incentive to continue using drugs.

A drug abuser may be simultaneously addicted to more than one substance. For instance, he may use amphetamines to stimulate himself or increase his physical performance and barbiturates to relax. Or he may follow cocaine use with heroin to moderate cocaine's stimulant effect. Such experimentation can be dangerous, particularly if the person uses synergistic drugs, such as barbiturates and alcohol. It also complicates assessment and intervention because the person may be experiencing withdrawal from several drugs at the same time.

## Causes of substance abuse

No single theory explains what causes substance abuse. Rather, evidence points to a combination of influences: psychological, familial, cultural, environmental, and biological.

*Psychological causes.* The typical substance abuser — anxious, angry, overly dependent, and depressed — has lowered self-esteem. The effect of alcohol or other drugs may provide a false sense of control and power over the source of his conflict. It also may create new areas of conflict resulting from guilt, fear of discovery, and the impact of the abused substance on the person's biopsychosocial function.

*Familial causes.* A dysfunctional family background may interfere with normal psychological and emotional development. Dysfunctional families commonly lack stability, have violent interactions with others, and have difficulty communicating. Such families tend to be distrustful of society and have histories of multigenerational addictive behavior. Relatives of alcoholics have a much greater risk of developing alcoholism than the general population. Children of alcoholics may become alcoholics themselves, even though many are repelled by their parents' behavior. Some patients may have a genetic predisposition toward drug and alcohol abuse.

*Cultural causes.* A person's cultural background and social interactions can influence his acceptance of drug and alcohol use. For instance, certain cultural, religious, and ethnic groups encourage alcohol use to celebrate an important event. As well, peer pressure may cause a person to acquire values that promote substance abuse.

Advertising supports society's message of using alcohol or other drugs to help relieve everyday stress. Ambivalence about alcohol and drug use compounds the problem. For instance, a parent may try to teach his child about the dangers of drug use while he continues to drink alcohol himself.

Society views substance abuse differently, depending on the substance being abused, the person abusing it, and the setting or context in which the abuse takes place. For instance, an executive who has several cocktails at lunch and can't accomplish much work in the afternoon isn't usually regarded as a substance abuser. However, a secretary who keeps a bottle of vodka in her desk drawer and drinks it during work would probably be counseled to seek help for alcohol abuse.

*Environmental causes.* A person who lives in an environment where drugs are easily accessible runs a higher risk of becoming a substance abuser. The risk becomes even greater if several members of his peer group abuse drugs or alcohol.

***Biological causes.*** Some people may have a chemical deficiency that predisposes them to become substance abusers.

## Challenges in patient care

To provide effective, compassionate care to a chemically dependent patient, you must first examine your own feelings about addiction. Identifying your attitudes and prejudices about alcohol and drug abuse can help you deal honestly and objectively with the patient and his family.

Examine how you communicate with alcoholics and drug abusers, checking for judgmental, moralistic, or patronizing comments. Identify any tendency to assume a destructive role, such as persecutor (being punitive), victim (allowing the patient to blame, use, or manipulate you), or enabler (accepting responsibility for the patient's behavior). Once you've become aware of your feelings, acknowledge your limitations and seek appropriate assistance when caring for such patients. Enlist the help of a psychiatric clinical nurse specialist or a psychiatrist when appropriate.

***Realistic approach.*** Work to develop a positive attitude about helping any chemically dependent patient. But don't expect complete success. Relapses occur, no matter what you do or how hard you try. This may not be your patient's first attempt to break his drug or alcohol addiction, so give him encouragement and emphasize his progress.

***Dual-diagnosis patient.*** You may encounter a patient who has a dual diagnosis: at least one form of chemical dependence accompanied by a major mental illness, such as a psychotic, mood, or anxiety disorder. Such a patient must be free from his chemical dependence before being treated for his mental illness. Unfortunately, few health care institutions are prepared to meet the special treatment needs of dual-diagnosis patients.

# Assessment

When you assess a patient for substance abuse, look for either acute intoxication or chronic abuse. An acutely intoxicated patient may also have a preexisting problem with chronic abuse. Be sure to assess for chronic abuse after the acute stage or physical illness has been treated.

## Acute alcohol intoxication

Most patients don't seek medical help for acute alcohol intoxication. Usually, they're brought to the hospital because they've been involved in a car accident or because someone found them showing signs of acute intoxication.

***History.*** Because the patient probably will be unable to provide accurate information, obtain his present history from whoever brings him to the hospital. Try to find out how much and what type of alcohol he had to drink. When was his last drink? Does he use alcohol often, or was this his first time? In many cases, adolescents who've never drunk alcohol before ingest large amounts and are brought to the hospital for respiratory depression or coma. Also determine if the patient is taking any medications that can exacerbate the effects of alcohol. (See *Reviewing drug-alcohol interactions,* page 190.)

If the patient can talk, ask him

## Reviewing drug-alcohol interactions

| DRUG | DRUG-ALCOHOL EFFECTS |
|---|---|
| Analgesics<br>Antianxiety drugs<br>Antidepressants<br>Antihistamines<br>Antipsychotics<br>Hypnotics | Deepened central nervous system (CNS) depression |
| Monoamine oxidase<br>inhibitors | Deepened CNS depression; possible hypertensive crisis wth some<br>types of beer and high-tyramine-content wines (Chianti, Alicante) |
| Oral antidiabetics | Disulfiram-like effects (facial flushing, headache), especially with<br>chlorpropamide; possible increased antidiabetic activity if food in-<br>take isn't adequate |
| Some antibacterial<br>agents (cephalo-<br>sporins, metronida-<br>zole) | Disulfiram-like effects |

about his recent alcohol use in a tolerant, nonthreatening way. Be prepared for insults and threats. Try to avoid direct eye contact for more than a few seconds because an intoxicated patient may interpret this as a challenge.

*Physical examination.* Check for physical signs and symptoms suggesting alcohol use. A patient with *mild to moderate intoxication* will have fruity breath odor or breath that smells of alcohol, diminished motor coordination, dysmetria, ataxia, nystagmus, blurred vision, flushed face, orthostatic hypotension, and possibly hematemesis. He also may be loud and boisterous, and his mood may quickly change from quiet to violent. Or he may be stuporous.

A patient with *severe intoxication* may exhibit decreased respiratory rate, slow pulse rate, low blood pressure, sluggish reflexes, and low body temperature. Severe intoxica-

tion can lead to shock and coma. A blood alcohol level above 0.1%, or 100 mg/dl, confirms acute intoxication. (See *How alcohol levels can affect behavior.*)

### Chronic alcohol abuse
If you suspect chronic alcohol abuse or if your patient is in a high-risk group for alcoholism, investigate the extent of his dependence and its effect on his daily life. Rarely is a patient aware that he's developing a problem with alcoholism. Instead, he'll typically use defense mechanisms—denial, rationalization, and projection—that help protect him from reality. This can make it difficult to obtain an accurate history.

*History.* Ask the patient about his daily alcohol use, including type, quantity, and frequency. Like many patients who chronically abuse alcohol, he'll probably tell you how much and how often he drinks, but he may deny that his drinking is out of control or disrupting his personal and professional life. He may downplay the impact alcohol has on his life. Or he may simply state that he can't imagine getting through the day without drinking. You may want to use an assessment tool, such as the Michigan Alcoholism Screening Test, to help determine if the patient has a problem with alcoholism. (See *Performing an alcohol screening test,* page 192.)

*General observations.* During the health history interview, observe the patient's manner in answering questions about alcohol. A guarded or hostile reply may be your first clue to chronic abuse. Also, check the patient's breath odor for alcohol or mouthwash.

*Defense mechanisms.* Note whether the patient uses a defense mechanism, such as rationalization, to cover up or deny his alcohol problem. His reasons for drinking may vary or even appear contradictory. For instance, he may state that he was drinking to celebrate a daughter's wedding or to mourn a friend's death, because of sickness or good health, because it's rainy or it's sunny.

A patient who uses projection as a defense mechanism may transfer his own feelings of guilt, inadequacy, and low self-esteem onto you. If he feels that you regard him as worthless, he may respond to you with anger and hostility. By understanding his reason for using the defense mechanism, you can avoid responding with hurt, bewilderment, or anger.

*Motivation for change.* Try to assess the patient's willingness to stop drinking. Even when a patient wants to gain control over his alco-

## How alcohol levels can affect behavior

This list shows how your patient's behavior may reflect the amount of alcohol in his bloodstream.
☐ Blood alcohol levels up to 0.1% (100 mg/dl) may produce decreased inhibitions, loud speech, and silliness.
☐ Blood alcohol levels between 0.1% and 0.2% may produce decreased coordination, impaired memory, moodiness, shortened attention span, slurred speech, and unsteady gait.
☐ Blood alcohol levels between 0.2% and 0.3% may produce ataxia, irritability, stupor, and tremor.
☐ Blood alcohol levels above 0.3% may produce unconsciousness.

holism, the task can be overwhelming. But when he hasn't identified the need to change his behavior, it's impossible.

***Physical examination.*** Chronic alcohol ingestion affects almost every body tissue. Tissue damage results from the direct, irritating effects of alcohol on the body; changes that take place in the body during the metabolism of alcohol; malnutrition; aggravation of existing disease; accidents that occur while intoxicated; and noncompliance with medical treatment while drinking.

*Physical complaints.* Assess any physical complaints that may stem from chronic alcohol abuse. For example, patients who chronically abuse alcohol are more prone to accidental injuries, for which they may delay seeking treatment for 24 hours or more. They also carry a higher risk of infection, malaise, dyspepsia, cigarette burns on the fingers, and fractures.

## Performing an alcohol screening test

Several assessment tools, such as the 1971 Michigan Alcoholism Screening Test (shown here) and the shorter version of the test developed in 1975, can help pinpoint the nature and severity of your patient's alcohol abuse. To use this test, ask your patient the following questions. For each positive response (except where indicated), score the number of points shown in the right column; then total the points. Generally, a score of five or more points indicates alcoholism; a score of four points suggests alcoholism; and a score of three or fewer points indicates that the patient isn't an alcoholic.

| Questions | Points |
|---|---|
| 1. Do you feel you are a normal drinker? (By normal, we mean do you drink less than or as much as most other people?)* | 2 |
| 2. Have you ever awakened the morning after drinking the night before and found that you could not remember a part of the evening? | 2 |
| 3. Does your spouse, a parent, or another near relative ever worry or complain about your drinking? | 1 |
| 4. Can you stop drinking without a struggle after one or two drinks?* | 2 |
| 5. Do you ever feel guilty about your drinking? | 1 |
| 6. Do friends or relatives think you are a normal drinker?* | 2 |
| 7. Are you able to stop drinking when you want to?* | 2 |
| 8. Have you ever attended a meeting of Alcoholics Anonymous (AA)? | 5 |
| 9. Have you gotten into physical fights when drinking? | 1 |
| 10. Has your drinking ever created problems between you and your spouse, a parent, or another near relative? | 2 |
| 11. Has your wife or husband (or another family member) ever gone to anyone for help about your drinking? | 2 |
| 12. Have you ever lost friends because of drinking? | 2 |
| 13. Have you ever gotten into trouble at work or school because you were drinking? | 2 |
| 14. Have you ever lost a job because of drinking? | 2 |
| 15. Have you ever neglected your obligations, your family, or your work for 2 or more days in a row because you were drinking? | 2 |
| 16. Do you drink before noon fairly often? | 1 |
| 17. Have you ever been told you have liver trouble? Cirrhosis? | 2 |
| 18. After heavy drinking have you ever had delirium tremens (DTs) or severe shaking, or heard voices or seen things that weren't really there?** | 2 |
| 19. Have you ever gone to anyone for help about your drinking? | 5 |
| 20. Have you ever been a patient in a psychiatric hospital or on a psychiatric ward of a general hospital where drinking was a part of the problem that resulted in hospitalization? | 5 |
| 21. Have you ever been seen at a psychiatric or mental health clinic, or gone to any doctor, social worker, or counselor, for help with any emotional problem where drinking was part of the problem? | 2 |
| 22. Have you ever been arrested for drunk driving, driving while intoxicated, or driving under the influence of alcoholic beverages? (If, yes, how many times? ____)† | 2 |
| 23. Have you ever been arrested or taken into custody, even for a few hours, because of other drunk behavior? (If yes, how many times? _____)† | 2 |

**Key**
* Alcoholic response is negative.
** Score five points for delirium tremens.
† Score two points for each arrest.

Adapted from Selzer, M.L. "The Michigan Alcoholism Screening Test: The Quest for a New Diagnostic Instrument," *American Journal of Psychiatry* 127(12):1653-58, June 1971.

*Skin changes.* Inspect the patient's skin for changes associated with chronic alcohol abuse. For instance, rosacea, telangiectasia, and rhinophyma accompany the vascular and nutritional changes that occur in chronic alcohol abuse. Palmar erythema is seen with chronic alcoholism. And spider angiomas are an early sign of alcohol-related liver disease.

*Fetal alcohol syndrome.* If the patient is a woman, determine if she's pregnant. Alcohol crosses the placental barrier and can cause fetal birth defects. Heavy drinking during pregnancy can cause fetal alcohol syndrome, resulting in growth deficiency, mental retardation, learning disabilities, organ problems, and distinct facial characteristics.

*Alcohol withdrawal.* If the patient has a history of regular alcohol use, examine him for indications of alcohol withdrawal. Initial symptoms include anorexia, nausea, anxiety, fever, insomnia, diaphoresis, and tremor. These may develop shortly after he stops drinking — when he enters the hospital, for instance. Alcohol withdrawal can last up to 7 days and may cause a variety of symptoms, ranging from mild disorientation to seizures. (See *Recognizing alcohol withdrawal,* page 194.)

Monitor the patient's vital signs, and be alert for elevated pulse rate (110 beats/minute or more) and blood pressure (150/90 mm Hg or higher). Also monitor the patient for the onset of generalized tonic-clonic seizures. (If the patient has a seizure, be sure to consider other causes, such as underlying head trauma, as well.)

*Alcohol withdrawal delirium.* If the patient is experiencing alcohol with-

drawal, monitor for the onset of delirium. This usually occurs 3 to 4 days after the patient stops drinking, but it can begin anytime between 1 and 5 days after he has his last drink. For more than 80% of patients, delirium lasts less than 3 days; for about 15% of patients, it lasts less than 24 hours.

Alcohol withdrawal delirium is characterized by disorientation to time and place, and a profoundly delirious state with severe tremulousness, agitation, and excessive motor activity. Visual or tactile hallucinations also may occur, causing panic and violent behavior. Increased autonomic nervous system activity may be marked by tachycardia, dilated pupils, and fever.

***Diagnostic tests.*** The doctor may order a serum alcohol level to determine the degree of intoxication. Breath test results should correlate with the serum alcohol level. More than 50% of chronic alcoholics show increased levels of serum gamma-glutamyltransferase. Alcoholic patients also commonly show increased mean corpuscular volume, reduced white blood cell count, and elevated serum levels of uric acid, triglycerides, aspartate aminotransferase (formerly SGOT), and urea.

Expect a patient experiencing alcohol withdrawal delirium to have nonspecific ST- and T-wave changes on the electrocardiogram (ECG). He'll probably have a normal EEG because of the absence of alcohol. Other diagnostic tests can determine the amount of alcohol-related tissue damage present. For instance, endoscopy may reveal esophageal varices, gastric ulcers, or gastritis.

### Acute drug intoxication
Most drug abusers use psychoactive drugs to achieve stimulant, hallucino-

## Recognizing alcohol withdrawal

Alcohol withdrawal affects your patient's motor control, mental status, and body functions. This list of signs and symptoms of alcohol withdrawal can help you determine whether he's experiencing mild, moderate, or severe withdrawal.

**Mild withdrawal**
• Hand tremor
• Mild restlessness and anxiety
• Restless sleep or insomnia
• Anorexia
• Nausea
• Oriented to time and place
• No hallucinations
• Tachycardia
• Normal or slightly elevated systolic blood pressure
• Slight sweating
• No seizures

**Moderate withdrawal**
• Visible tremulousness
• Obvious restlessness and anxiety
• Marked insomnia; nightmares
• Marked anorexia
• Nausea and vomiting
• Variable confusion
• Vague, transient hallucinations
• Pulse rate of 100 to 120 beats/minute
• Elevated systolic blood pressure
• Obvious sweating
• Possible seizures

**Severe withdrawal
(alcohol withdrawal syndrome)**
• Uncontrollable shaking
• Extreme restlessness and agitation
• Intense fear and anxiety

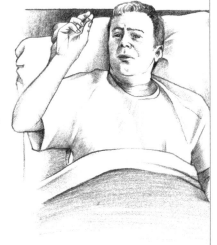

• Wakefulness
• Rejection of food and fluid except alcohol
• Dry heaves and vomiting
• Marked confusion and disorientation
• Frightening visual and occasional auditory hallucinations
• Pulse rate of 120 to 140 beats/minute
• Elevated systolic and diastolic blood pressure
• Marked hyperhydrosis
• Seizures

genic, or sedative effects. Different types of drugs produce different symptoms. (See *Reviewing commonly abused substances.*)

Typically, a patient won't seek medical attention for acute drug intoxication on his own. More likely, he'll be brought to the hospital by someone else for related physical problems, such as respiratory depression, altered level of conscious-

ness, injuries from a car accident, or burns from free-basing.

***History.*** If the patient's condition permits, ask which drugs he took, how much, and when. He may not answer your questions accurately because of drug-induced amnesia, a depressed level of consciousness, deliberate attempts to mislead or

*(Text continues on page 199.)*

# Reviewing commonly abused substances

| SUBSTANCE | SIGNS AND SYMPTOMS | INTERVENTIONS |
|---|---|---|
| **Stimulants** | | |
| **Cocaine**<br>• *Street names*: coke, flake, snow, nose candy, hits, crack (hardened form), rock, crank<br>• *Routes*: injection, speedballing (injection of both cocaine and heroin), sniffing, smoking (free-basing [with crack], smoking in cigarettes or glass water pipes)<br>• *Dependence*: psychological<br>• *Duration of effect*: 15 minutes to 2 hours; with crack, rapid "high" of short duration followed by down feeling<br>• *Medical uses*: local anesthetic | • *Use*: abdominal pain; alternating euphoria and apprehension; anorexia; cardiotoxicity, such as ventricular fibrillation; coma; confusion; diaphoresis; dilated pupils; fever; grandiosity; hallucinations; hyperpnea; hyperexcitability; hypotension or hypertension; insomnia; irritability; nausea and vomiting; pallor or cyanosis; perforated nasal septum with prolonged inhalation use; pressured speech; psychotic behavior with large doses; respiratory arrest; seizures; spasms; tachycardia; tachypnea; weight loss<br>• *Withdrawal*: anxiety, depression, fatigue | • Place patient in a quiet room.<br>• If cocaine was ingested, induce vomiting or perform gastric lavage; follow with activated charcoal and a saline cathartic.<br>• If cocaine was sniffed, use a cotton-tipped applicator to remove residual drug from mucous membranes.<br>• Monitor vital signs.<br>• Give propranolol for tachycardia.<br>• Give cardiopulmonary resuscitation for ventricular fibrillation and cardiac arrest, as indicated.<br>• Give a tepid sponge bath for fever.<br>• Give an anticonvulsant for seizures. |
| **Amphetamines**<br>• *Street names*: for amphetamine sulfate— bennies, grennies, cartwheels; for methamphetamine—speed, meth, crystal; for dextroamphetamine sulfate— dexies, hearts, oranges<br>• *Routes*: ingestion, injection<br>• *Dependence*: psychological<br>• *Duration of effect*: 1 to 4 hours<br>• *Medical uses*: hyperkinesis, narcolepsy, weight control | • *Use*: altered mental status (from confusion to paranoia), coma, diaphoresis, dilated reactive pupils, dry mouth, exhaustion, hallucinations, hyperactive deep tendon reflexes, hypertension, hyperthermia, paradoxical reaction in children, psychotic behavior with prolonged use, seizures, shallow respirations, tachycardia, tremors<br>• *Withdrawal*: abdominal tenderness, apathy, depression, disorientation, irritability, long periods of sleep, muscle aches, suicide (with sudden withdrawal) | • Place patient in a quiet room.<br>• If drug was ingested, induce vomiting or perform gastric lavage; follow with activated charcoal and a saline or magnesium sulfate cathartic.<br>• Add ammonium chloride or ascorbic acid to I.V. solution to acidify urine to a pH of 5.0<br>• Give mannitol to induce diuresis.<br>• Monitor vital signs.<br>• Give a short-acting barbiturate, such as pentobarbital, for seizures.<br>• Give haloperidol for violent behavior.<br>• Give phentolamine for hypertension.<br>• Give propranolol for tachyarrhythmias and lidocaine for ventricular arrhythmias.<br>• Restrain a hallucinating or paranoid patient.<br>• Give a tepid sponge bath for fever.<br>• Institute suicide precautions for withdrawal. |

*(continued)*

# Reviewing commonly abused substances (continued)

| SUBSTANCE | SIGNS AND SYMPTOMS | INTERVENTIONS |
|---|---|---|
| **Hallucinogens** | | |
| **Lysergic acid diethyl-amide (LSD)**<br>• *Street names:* acid, microdot, sugar, big D<br>• *Routes:* ingestion, smoking<br>• *Dependence:* possibly psychological<br>• *Duration of effect:* 8 to 12 hours<br>• *Medical uses:* none | • *Use:* abdominal cramps, arrhythmias, chills, depersonalization, diaphoresis, diarrhea, dilated pupils with overdose but constricted pupils with intoxication, distorted perception, dizziness, dry mouth, fever, grandiosity, hallucinations, heightened sense of awareness, hyperpnea, hypertension, illusions, increased salivation, muscle aches, mystical experiences, nausea, palpitations, seizures, tachycardia, vomiting<br>• *Withdrawal:* none | • Place patient in a quiet room.<br>• If drug was ingested, induce vomiting or perform gastric lavage; follow with activated charcoal and a cathartic.<br>• Give diazepam for seizures.<br>• Monitor vital signs.<br>• Reorient patient to time, place, and person.<br>• Restrain patient as needed. |
| **Phencyclidine**<br>• *Street names:* PCP, hog, angel dust, peace pill, crystal superjoint, elephant tranquilizer, rocket fuel<br>• *Routes:* ingestion, injection, smoking<br>• *Dependence:* possibly psychological<br>• *Duration of effect:* 30 minutes to days<br>• *Medical uses:* veterinary anesthetic | • *Use:* amnesia; blank stare; cardiac arrest; decreased awareness of surroundings; delusions; distorted body image; distorted sense of sight, hearing, and touch; drooling; euphoria; excitation and psychoses; fever; gait ataxia; hallucinations; hyperactivity; hypertensive crisis; individualized unpredictable effects; muscle rigidity; nystagmus; panic; poor perception of time and distance; possible chromosomal damage; psychotic behavior; recurrent coma; renal failure; seizures; sudden behavioral changes; tachycardia; violent behavior<br>• *Withdrawal:* none | • Place patient in a quiet room.<br>• If drug was ingested, induce vomiting or perform gastric lavage; follow with activated charcoal.<br>• Add ascorbic acid to I.V. solution to acidify urine. May need to acidify urine for up to 2 weeks because symptoms will reappear as fat cells release the drug.<br>• Monitor vital signs and hourly urine output.<br>• Give ordered diuretic.<br>• Give propranolol for hypertension or tachycardia; give nitroprusside for hypertensive crisis.<br>• Give diazepam for seizures.<br>• Give diazepam or haloperidol for agitation or psychotic behavior; give physostigmine salicylate, diazepam, chlordiazepoxide hydrochloride, or chlorpromazine hydrochloride for a "bad trip." |

## Reviewing commonly abused substances *(continued)*

| SUBSTANCE | SIGNS AND SYMPTOMS | INTERVENTIONS |
|---|---|---|
| **Depressants** | | |
| **Alcohol**<br>• *Found in:* beer, wine, distilled spirits; also contained in cough syrup, after-shave, and mouthwash<br>• *Route:* ingestion<br>• *Dependence:* physical, psychological<br>• *Duration of effect:* varies among persons and according to amount ingested; metabolized at a rate of 10 ml/hour<br>• *Medical uses:* neurolysis (absolute alcohol); emergency tocolytic; treatment of ethylene glycol and methanol poisoning | • *Acute use:* decreased inhibitions, euphoria followed by depression or hostility, impaired judgment, incoordination, respiratory depression, slurred speech, vomiting, unconsciousness, coma, death<br>• *Withdrawal:* delirium, hallucinations, seizures, tremor | • Place patient in a quiet room.<br>• If alcohol was ingested within 4 hours, induce vomiting or perform gastric lavage; follow with activated charcoal and a saline cathartic.<br>• Monitor vital signs and check for symptoms of withdrawal.<br>• Institute seizure precautions.<br>• Give diazepam for seizures.<br>• Give chlordiazepoxide, chloral hydrate, or paraldehyde for hallucinations and delirium.<br>• Provide I.V. fluid replacement as well as dextrose, thiamine, B-complex vitamins, and vitamin C to treat dehydration, hypoglycemia, and nutritional deficiencies.<br>• Assess lungs for signs of aspiration pneumonia.<br>• Prepare patient for dialysis if vital functions are severely depressed. |
| **Benzodiazepines (alprazolam, chlordiazepoxide hydrochloride, clonazepam, clorazepate dipotassium, diazepam, flurazepam, oxazepam, temazepam, triazolam)**<br>• *Street names:* vals, benzos<br>• *Routes:* ingestion, injection<br>• *Dependence:* physical, psychological<br>• *Duration of effect:* 4 to 8 hours<br>• *Medical uses:* antianxiety agent, anticonvulsant, sedative, hypnotic | • *Use:* ataxia, drowsiness, hypotension, increased self-confidence, relaxation, relief of anxiety, slurred speech<br>• *Overdose:* confusion, drowsiness, respiratory depression, coma, death<br>• *Withdrawal:* abdominal cramps, agitation, anxiety, diaphoresis, hypertension, tachycardia, tonic-clonic seizures, tremor, vomiting | • If drug was ingested, induce vomiting or perform gastric lavage; follow with activated charcoal and a cathartic.<br>• Monitor vital signs.<br>• Give supplemental oxygen for hypoxia-induced seizures.<br>• Give I.V. fluids for hypertension.<br>• Give physostigmine salicylate for respiratory or central nervous system (CNS) depression. |

*(continued)*

# Reviewing commonly abused substances (continued)

| SUBSTANCE | SIGNS AND SYMPTOMS | INTERVENTIONS |
|---|---|---|
| **Depressants** (continued) | | |
| **Barbiturates (amobarbital, phenobarbital, secobarbital)**<br>• *Street names*: for barbiturates – downers, sleepers, barbs; for amobarbital – blue angels, blue devils, bluebirds; for phenobarbital – phennies, purple hearts, goofballs; for secobarbital – reds, red devils, seccy<br>• *Routes*: ingestion, injection<br>• *Dependence*: physical, psychological<br>• *Duration*: 1 to 16 hours<br>• *Medical uses*: anesthetic, anticonvulsant, sedative, hypnotic | • *Use*: absent reflexes, blisters or bullous lesions, cyanosis, depressed level of consciousness (from confusion to coma), fever, flaccid muscles, hypotension, hypothermia, nystagmus, paradoxical reaction in children and elderly patients, poor pupil reaction to light, respiratory depression<br>• *Withdrawal*: agitation, anxiety, fever, insomnia, postural hypotension, tachycardia, tremor<br>• *Rapid withdrawal*: anorexia, apprehension, hallucinations, postural hypotension, tonic-clonic seizures, tremor, weakness | • If drug was ingested within 4 hours, induce vomiting or perform gastric lavage; follow with activated charcoal and a saline cathartic.<br>• Monitor vital signs and perform frequent neurologic and respiratory assessments.<br>• Give I.V. fluid bolus for hypotension.<br>• Give sodium bicarbonate after phenobarbital overdose to alkalinize urine and speed drug elimination.<br>• Monitor for evidence of withdrawal.<br>• Institute seizure precautions and protect patient from withdrawal.<br>• Use hypothermia or hyperthermia blanket for temperature alterations. |
| **Opiates (codeine, heroin, meperidine, morphine, opium)**<br>• *Street names*: for heroin – boy, junk, horse, H, smack, scag, stuff; for morphine – morph<br>• *Routes*: for codeine, meperidine, and morphine – ingestion, injection, smoking; for heroin – ingestion, injection, inhalation, smoking; for opium – ingestion, smoking<br>• *Dependence*: physical, psychological<br>• *Duration of effect*: 3 to 6 hours<br>• *Medical uses*: for codeine – analgesia, antitussive; for heroin – under investigation; for meperidine and morphine – analgesia; for opium – analgesia, antidiarrheal | • *Use*: analgesia, anorexia, arrhythmias, clammy skin, constipation, constricted pupils, decreased level of consciousness, detachment from reality, drowsiness, euphoria, hypotension, impaired judgment, increased pigmentation over veins, lack of concern, lethargy, nausea, needle marks, relaxation, respiratory depression, seizures, shallow breathing, skin lesions or abscesses, slow respirations, slurred speech, swollen or perforated nasal mucosa, thrombosed veins, urine retention, vomiting<br>• *Withdrawal*: abdominal cramps, anorexia, chills, diaphoresis, dilated pupils, hyperactive bowel sounds, irritability, nausea, panic, piloerection, runny nose, sweating, tremor, watery eyes, yawning | • If drug was ingested, induce vomiting or perform gastric lavage.<br>• Give naloxone until CNS effects are reversed.<br>• For overdose, give I.V. fluids to increase circulatory volume, assess lung sounds to monitor for evidence of pulmonary edema, and use extra blankets for hypothermia; if ineffective, use hyperthermia blanket.<br>• Reorient the patient to time, place, and person.<br>• Monitor for signs of withdrawal. |

## Reviewing commonly abused substances *(continued)*

| SUBSTANCE | SIGNS AND SYMPTOMS | INTERVENTIONS |
|---|---|---|
| **Cannabinoid** | | |
| **Marijuana**<br>• *Street names:* pot, grass, weed, Mary Jane, roach, reefer, joint, smoke, THC<br>• *Routes:* ingestion, smoking<br>• *Dependence:* physical<br>• *Duration of effect:* 2 to 3 hours<br>• *Medical uses:* antiemetic for chemotherapy | • *Use:* acute psychosis, altered thinking processes, amotivational syndrome in chronic users, anxiety, bronchitis and asthma in chronic smokers, conjunctival reddening, decreased blood pressure when standing, decreased muscle strength, delusions, distorted sense of time and self-perception, dry mouth, euphoria, extreme agitation, hallucinations, impaired cognitive ability, impaired short-term memory, incoordination, increased hunger, increased sense of well-being, increased systolic pressure when supine, keen sense of hearing, mood impairment, panic, paranoia, relaxation, respiratory depression, spontaneous laughter, tachycardia, vivid visual imagery<br>• *Withdrawal:* chills, decreased appetite, fever, insomnia, irritability, nervousness, rebound increase in rapid-eye-movement sleep, restlessness, tremor, weight loss | • Place patient in a quiet room.<br>• Monitor vital signs.<br>• Give supplemental oxygen for respiratory depression.<br>• Give I.V. fluids for hypotension.<br>• Give diazepam for extreme agitation and acute psychosis. |

misinform, or ignorance about the type of drug taken. If so, ask someone who was with the patient at the time, if possible. Because of the legal issues surrounding drug use, you may not receive reliable information. If possible, check the patient's possessions for evidence of drug paraphernalia.

***Physical examination.*** Because substance abuse commonly causes severe respiratory depression and can have cardiotoxic effects, you must first assess the patient's airway, breathing, and circulation. Keep oxygen, suction equipment, and emergency airway equipment nearby, and be prepared to intervene immediately if his status deteriorates.

Check the patient's vital signs for possible indications of shock, such as decreased blood pressure and a faint, rapid pulse. Note whether he has any obvious signs of trauma, such as burns, bruises, or lacerations. Check his extremities for needle marks, suggesting I.V. drug use.

## Chronic drug abuse

Typically, a chronic drug abuser comes into frequent contact with the health care system because of related physiologic crises. The crises may stem from overdose, physical deterioration due to illness or malnutrition, or substance withdrawal.

*History.* Try to determine which drugs the patient takes, how much, and when. Review his psychosocial history to detect behavior patterns that suggest drug use or an increased risk of using drugs. Legal and social problems associated with drug use may make the patient unwilling to provide reliable information. Also, the patient may not consider his drug use a problem. If possible, question the patient's family members or friends about behaviors that may suggest a drug problem.

*Medical history.* Find out about the patient's past and present illnesses, including hepatitis and HIV infection, which may be transmitted by sharing I.V. needles. If the patient is a woman, ask about drug-related amenorrhea. If she's pregnant, assess her knowledge of the harmful effects of drug abuse on fetal development.

*Medical care patterns.* Also find out about the patient's medical care history. When and how often does he seek medical care? Keep in mind that he may be using a real or imagined medical problem to obtain drugs. Be alert for the patient who:
• feigns intense pain or illness, such as migraine headache, myocardial infarction, or renal colic, to obtain analgesics
• claims an allergy to milder analgesics to get stronger narcotics
• asks for a specific medication and

has a good working knowledge of pharmacology
• has a history of overdose or a high tolerance for drug doses
• claims a chronic injury or illness but refuses a diagnostic workup.

*Psychosocial history.* Check several forms of identification to verify the patient's name and address. Is the hospital one that a person from his area is likely to use? If not, he may be avoiding hospitals closer to his home, where he's known as a drug seeker.

Try to determine how the patient views his drug use. Does he feel that drugs are causing problems in his life? Does he think he's addicted to drugs? Also determine the patient's motivation for change. Does he feel the need to change his addictive patterns? As with alcohol, giving up drugs is extremely difficult at best, but when the patient doesn't acknowledge his problems or the need to change, the task becomes impossible.

*General observations.* During the health history interview, observe the patient's behavior for characteristics of chronic drug abuse. Typically, a chronic drug abuser is disruptive, demanding, and anxious. He may experience dramatic mood swings, impaired memory, and flashbacks. Slurred speech, depression, violent acts, and thought disorders are also common.

Monitor the patient for attempts to obtain drugs from visiting family members or friends, staff members, or his roommate. He may use bribery, threats, coercion, or manipulation. He also may try to play off one staff member against another, a technique called "staff splitting." This can result in conflict among staff members and inconsistent care.

***Physical examination.*** Depending on the nature of the patient's drug abuse, he may appear reasonably healthy or obviously drugged on initial assessment. Physical findings can be directly related to the drug use or associated with disorders caused by drug use.

First, check for indications of drug overdose. Depending on what type of drug the patient took, he may exhibit signs of CNS depression, ranging from lethargy to coma; signs of CNS stimulation, ranging from euphoria to assaultive behavior; hallucinations; respiratory depression; seizure activity; nausea; vomiting; and rigor (severe chills).

Check the patient's vital signs, noting any fever. Fever can be a direct effect of intoxication with a CNS stimulant or a hallucinogen. It also can occur with CNS depressant withdrawal and infection from I.V. drug use.

As the patient's condition permits, perform a head-to-toe physical examination.

*Eyes, nose, and mouth.* You may see lacrimation and rhinorrhea from opiate withdrawal, nystagmus from CNS depressant or PCP intoxication, and drooping eyelids from opiate or CNS depressant use. Check the patient's pupil reaction. You'll see constricted pupils with opiate use or withdrawal, and dilated pupils with the use of hallucinogens or amphetamines.

Also check the patient's nose and mouth. Erythematous, atrophied, or perforated nasal mucosa may result from drug sniffing. Dental problems associated with poor oral hygiene may stem from chronic drug use. Also inspect under the tongue for evidence that the patient is using the veins there as I.V. drug injection sites.

*Skin.* Note whether the patient is diaphoretic. Sweating commonly indicates intoxication with opiates or CNS stimulants and most drug withdrawal syndromes.

Check the patient's extremities for needle marks, suggesting I.V. drug use. Also check for tracks along veins, caused by deposits of carbon after injection with a needle that has been flamed before use. Tattoo marks may be used to obscure or disguise injection sites or tracks. Be sure to check less obvious injection sites, such as under the nails and the veins of the breasts and penis.

Also observe the skin for signs of drug-related trauma or changes. You may detect excoriation from compulsive scratching, or cellulitis from self-injection. Because chronic drug use depresses the patient's immune response, making him more vulnerable to infection, you may note abscesses at injection sites. You also may note swollen hands — a late indication of thrombophlebitis or fascial infection caused by self-injection into the hands or arms.

*Respiratory status.* Be alert for signs of respiratory depression, especially if your patient may have taken a drug overdose. Pulmonary edema can result from the sudden drop in blood pressure that may occur in an overdose. Aspiration pneumonia can be caused by the vomiting and loss of gag reflex that commonly occur in a drug overdose. When you auscultate the patient's lungs, note any bilateral crackles and rhonchi — common complications of any drug that's smoked or inhaled and a possible indication of opiate overdose.

*Cardiovascular status.* Monitor your patient's blood pressure. You may detect acute-onset hypertension unresponsive to treatment in a patient who has taken an overdose of a CNS stimulant or some hallucinogens. You may find hypotension in a patient who has taken an overdose of a CNS depressant or an opiate, or in one who's in the late stage of a severe withdrawal reaction. Also monitor the patient's cardiac rhythm and rate. You may detect cardiac arrhythmias in a patient who has taken an overdose of a CNS stimulant or some hallucinogens, or in one who's experiencing withdrawal from CNS depressants or opiates.

*Abdomen.* Palpate and percuss the patient's abdomen. Abdominal pain (cramping) is common during opiate withdrawal. An enlarged liver with or without tenderness may be secondary to hepatitis caused by alcoholism or I.V. drug abuse. Hemorrhoids are a common consequence of the constipating effects of opiate usage.

*Neurologic status.* Check for drug-induced effects on the patient's neurologic system. Examples include tremor, hyperreflexia, hyporeflexia, peripheral neuropathy, seizures, organic brain syndrome, Wernicke's encephalopathy, and Korsakoff's syndrome.

**Diagnostic tests.** You'll get definitive information about your patient's substance abuse after the results of initial toxicology screening are available. Blood tests for toxicology identify the presence and serum level of the drugs used.

If the patient has drug-related hepatitis, additional blood tests may show elevated serum globulin levels, hypoglycemia, leukocytosis, liver function abnormalities, elevated mean corpuscular hemoglobin (MCH), elevated mean corpuscular volume (MCV), elevated uric acid levels, and decreased blood urea nitrogen levels. If he has syphilis, he also may have positive results on the Venereal Disease Research Laboratory (VDRL) or rapid plasma reagin tests. And if he has been infected with the HIV virus, he'll test positive for HIV infection.

The patient's chest X-rays may reveal multiple pulmonary foreign body granulomas, resulting from abuse of drugs that have been processed with talc, cellulose, or similar foreign material. You may also see evidence of multiple rib fractures in varying degrees of healing — the result of frequent falls by the chronically intoxicated patient.

# Intervention

Most forms of therapy share the same goal: to stop substance abuse and to treat its physiologic, neurologic, and psychological effects. The specific interventions you'll take depend on whether your patient abuses alcohol or other drugs and whether his condition is acute or chronic. Medications, behavior modification, counseling, and other forms of therapy can all play a role in the patient's overall treatment plan. As the patient's condition indicates, treatment may range from providing basic life support to planning a rehabilitation program.

## Acute alcohol intoxication
Treatment of acute alcohol intoxication involves monitoring the patient's vital signs and ECG, and checking his neurologic status as ordered. It also includes treating alcohol's physiologic effects and calming or restraining the patient as needed.

*Emergency interventions.* If the patient's level of consciousness is altered, take precautions to prevent aspiration. Replace fluids as needed; severe diaphoresis may increase fluid requirements. As ordered, obtain a blood sample for serum glucose analysis, and give I.V. glucose to prevent a hypoglycemic reaction.

Alcoholism can induce vitamin deficiencies and starvation ketoacidosis. As ordered, give thiamine to prevent Wernicke's encephalopathy. Assess and correct any associated disorders, such as hypothermia, acidosis, infection, trauma, or GI bleeding.

*Medication therapy.* Administer a benzodiazepine (diazepam, diazepoxide, lorazepam, or oxazepam), as ordered, if you need to sedate the patient to forestall severe withdrawal reactions. Continue giving the medication until the patient becomes manageable. As the patient's vital signs stabilize, the doctor will decrease the sedative dosage gradually over 3 to 5 days. Then he'll discontinue the drug. Observe the patient's physical condition and behavior for adverse effects and possible toxicity from the substitute drug.

*Calm atmosphere.* When caring for the patient, approach him in a nonthreatening manner. Avoid sustained eye contact, and try to listen to what he says, even if he becomes verbally abusive. Request help from other staff members or security personnel if the patient becomes aggressive or threatening. If necessary, physically restrain the patient according to hospital policy.

Promote a calm atmosphere and, if the patient's condition permits, allow him to sleep off the effects of the alcohol. Try to keep the patient oriented should he become confused or have hallucinations.

## Chronic alcohol abuse

Interventions include medication therapy, behavior modification, family counseling, referral to support groups, and patient teaching.

*Medications.* If the patient's alcohol problem is severe, the doctor may order disulfiram therapy as part of an overall treatment plan. Disulfiram helps prevent impulsive drinking by sensitizing the patient to alcohol and causing an aversive physiologic response if he uses alcohol in any form.

*Patient preparation.* To prepare the patient for disulfiram therapy, make sure he understands the purpose, procedure, and precautions for using the drug. After he takes the drug, he must avoid drinking alcohol. Explain that using alcohol while taking disulfiram can cause severe headache, nausea and vomiting, flushing, hypotension, tachycardia, dyspnea, diaphoresis, chest pain, palpitations, dizziness, and confusion. In some patients, it also can lead to respiratory and cardiac collapse, unconsciousness, seizures, and death. To prevent a negative reaction, stress the need to avoid all alcohol and alcohol-containing products. These include cough medicines, rubbing compounds, vinegar, after-shave lotions, and some mouthwashes. Disulfiram will work up to 14 days after the patient takes his last dose.

*Behavior modification.* This form of therapy involves teaching the patient how to stop using defense mechanisms, such as denial, projection, and rationalization, that enable him to continue drinking. Depending on the nature of his alcoholism, the patient may benefit from individual, family, or group counseling. The patient's perception of his problem and his motivation to change will determine his success with rehabilitation.

*Patient preparation.* To prepare the patient for behavior modification therapy, help improve his self-esteem so that he can learn to meet his needs without relying on alcohol. Promote measures to enhance self-esteem, such as providing tasks that lead to success (such as volunteering), exploring areas of competence (such as hobbies and skills the patient has), and allowing the patient to express hope for sobriety. Identify ways to cope with loneliness other than drinking alcohol. Explore methods of relieving tension and anxiety and developing constructive coping skills to avoid frustration.

Help the patient accept that some of his problems result from drinking and that he must stop all alcohol and drug intake. Confront him about his behavior, and allow him to express his rationalizations. Then help him explore the real reasons behind his drinking.

*Family counseling.* Assess the family's ability to cope with the patient's alcoholism. Family members, confused by the patient's erratic behavior, are subject to the same feelings of guilt, depression, loneliness, and low self-esteem as the alcoholic and often use the same defense mechanisms. They may act in ways that sustain rather than change the drinking behavior. Involve both the patient and his family in the treatment plan to increase their understanding of alcoholism.

*Support groups.* Refer the patient and his family to an appropriate support group. For instance, Alcoholics Anonymous (AA), a self-help group composed of recovering alcoholics, believes that mutual support can give the alcoholic strength to abstain from alcohol and other substance abuse.

Family support groups promote the message that family members aren't responsible for, and can't control, the alcoholic's drinking but can still live meaningful, purposeful lives. Al-Anon is a self-help group that meets the needs of spouses and loved-ones of alcoholics. Alateen addresses the concerns of adolescents who are involved with alcoholic family members. Adult Children of Alcoholics meets the needs of adults with alcoholic parents.

*Patient teaching.* Inform the patient and his family about the possibility of relapse, and establish an appropriate care plan. Negotiate the plan's terms with the patient and his family so that family members won't feel ambivalent about instituting the plan.

To help prevent a relapse, teach the patient and his family about the over-the-counter and prescription medications that contain alcohol. Medications containing as little as 3.8% alcohol can evoke behavioral responses, such as irritability, restlessness, indifference, anxiety, depression, and active avoidance of interpersonal contacts.

## Acute drug intoxication

Treatment of acute drug overdose begins with basic life support. After you've stabilized your patient's vital functions, continue to treat related symptoms and complications, as indicated.

*Emergency interventions.* Assess the patient's airway, breathing, and circulation. Keep emergency equipmont nearby. As ordered, give the patient naloxone to reverse narcotic effects. Monitor his vital signs and ECG readings, and perform frequent neurologic assessments.

Institute seizure precautions to protect the patient from injury if seizures occur during substance withdrawal. As with all patients, practice universal precautions to protect yourself from contracting a blood-borne illness associated with I.V. drug use.

If indicated, take appropriate steps to stop further absorption of the abused substance. These steps may include using gastric lavage, activated charcoal, forced diuresis to either alkalinize or acidify the urine, and possibly hemoperfusion and hemodialysis.

Obtain samples of blood, urine, and vomitus for toxicology screening and analysis. Don't delay treatment because results may take several hours to process.

***Symptomatic interventions.*** A patient who abuses drugs can develop a multitude of symptoms and health problems related to his addiction. Provide appropriate treatment and support. For example, give a tachycardic patient a beta blocker or a calcium channel blocker, as ordered, to slow down his heart rate.

Provide one-on-one supervision for the patient, if necessary. Drug withdrawal sometimes results in aggressive behavior or frightening hallucinations. Orient the patient to person, place, time, and situation, and reorient him as needed to decrease any fear and confusion. Use restraints, if necessary, to prevent the patient from harming himself or others. Provide a quiet, calm environment with minimal stimulation to avoid agitating the patient.

## Chronic drug abuse

After you've intervened to correct acute intoxication or withdrawal, initiate measures to rehabilitate the patient. Such measures may include monitoring behavior, establishing a therapeutic nurse-patient relationship, medication therapy, psychotherapy, and patient teaching.

Successful rehabilitation hinges on the patient's ability to replace his need for drugs with other, more positive life goals. It's almost impossible to rehabilitate a patient who'll be returning to the same social environment and stresses that created the dependence. When planning a rehabilitation program, consider the patient's motivation for change, available support systems, and community resources.

***Behavior monitoring.*** While the patient is hospitalized, make sure he understands the hospital's standards for acceptable behavior. Observe his behavior and its effect on the staff. As with chronic alcoholics, chronic drug abusers will use manipulation, bribery, and other means to obtain drugs. If conflicts among staff members result, consult with a psychiatric clinical nurse specialist to develop a consistent care plan that sets definite limits for the patient.

***Therapeutic relationship.*** Gain the patient's trust by establishing a therapeutic nurse-patient relationship. If the patient feels free to discuss his drug dependence, you may be able to help him confront his problem and begin the rehabilitation process. If the patient denies that he has a drug problem, try to discuss the reality of his drug use and its effect on his life.

Try to determine any underlying problems that may have precipitated his drug dependence. For in-

## Finding help

**Toll-free national hotlines**
*National Parents' Resource Institute for Drug Abuse (PRIDE) Drug Information Services*
1-800-67-PRIDE

*National Cocaine Hotline*
1-800-COCAINE

*National Institute on Drug Abuse Cocaine Hotline*
1-800-662-HELP

**Other information sources**
*Families in Action National Drug Information Center*
2296 Henderson Mill Rd., Suite 204
Atlanta, GA 30345

*National Clearinghouse for Alcohol and Drug Abuse Information*
P.O. Box 416
Kensington, MD 20795

*National Federation of Parents for Drug-Free Youth*
8730 Georgia Ave., Suite 200
Silver Spring, MD 20910

*Narcotics Anonymous*
P.O. Box 9999
Van Nuys, CA 91409

stance, the patient may drive other people away by being overly dependent on them, thus increasing his dependence on drugs.

Seek ways to help the patient overcome his dependence — for instance, by increasing his self-esteem. Identify the patient's strengths, and help him find options to use his talents in positive ways. During hospitalization, make sure the patient's hygiene needs are met. If he looks and feels well cared for, he'll feel better about himself.

If the patient expresses anger, let

him know you understand, but set appropriate limits. For instance, allow him to express his anger but not to harm himself or others. Provide diversions to channel his anger, if needed.

***Medication therapy.*** The doctor may order methadone therapy in conjunction with behavior modification techniques. Oral doses of methadone don't produce the euphoria associated with other opiates, but they do satisfy the patient's physiologic need for the drug and prevent withdrawal symptoms. An overdose may occur if the patient obtains additional methadone from another source — the black market, for instance.

Narcotic antagonists block or antagonize opiates, preventing them from acting. Treatment succeeds only if the patient is highly motivated to eliminate his drug dependence. A short duration of action enables the patient to experience the full effects of opiates one day after failure to take a narcotic antagonist.

***Psychotherapy.*** Consult with a psychiatric clinical nurse specialist or a psychiatrist to help plan an effective rehabilitation program and provide access to community support services. The program may include individual, family, or group therapy.

*Individual therapy* provides a nonjudgmental setting in which the patient can explore his problems and find solutions. He'll learn ways to deal with his dependence, low self-esteem, manipulative behavior, and anger.

*Family therapy* actively involves family members in identifying and changing behavior patterns that trigger drug use.

*Group therapy* allows the patient's peers to help him confront his problem and deal with the realities of peer pressure

**Patient teaching.** If the patient isn't willing to accept drug rehabilitation, you'll need to teach him how to prevent associated injury and complications.

Explain how HIV infection and hepatitis are transmitted by exchanging body fluids, as occurs during unprotected intercourse or when sharing I.V. needles with other drug users. Teach him to use a new needle for each injection or to clean used needles first with a solution of chlorine bleach and water. Encourage him to use a condom each time he has intercourse. If your patient is a woman, explain the effects of drug use on the fetus and discuss contraception. Finally, provide the patient with a list of resources so that he'll know whom to contact if he decides to seek help. (See *Finding help.*)

# Evaluation

Addiction is a chronic condition, and recovery is an ongoing process. So determining the success of your interventions isn't as straightforward as it is with certain physical problems. Depending on the patient's condition, success could be something as simple as getting him to trust you.

## Recovery process
Chronic substance abusers typically experience relapses. So an evaluation of the ongoing recovery process must be based on realistic expectations of treatment goals.

A counselor may determine whether the patient is abstaining from alcohol and other drugs and whether he and his family are using effective communication techniques to decrease anxiety and conflict. The counselor may also find out if behavior modification techniques are helping.

A counselor may evaluate how the patient's substance abuse affects his ongoing health. Is he still suffering from the physiologic effects of substance abuse, or have interventions corrected his physical complaints? Also, the counselor will try to determine the patient's commitment to living a life free of alcohol and other drugs. Without a strong motivation, complete rehabilitation is impossible.

## Suggested readings

*Diagnostic and Statistical Manual of Mental Disorders,* 3rd ed., revised. Washington, D.C.: American Psychiatric Association, 1987.

Gilman, A.G., et al., eds. *Goodman and Gilman's The Pharmacological Basis of Therapeutics,* 8th ed. New York: Pergamon Press, 1990.

Grinspoon, L., and Bakalar, J.B. "Drug Dependence: Nonnarcotic Agents," in *Comprehensive Textbook of Psychiatry,* vol. 1, 5th ed. Edited by Kaplan, H.I., and Sadock, B.J. Baltimore: Williams & Wilkins Co., 1989.

Pasquali, E.A., et al. *Mental Health Nursing, A Holistic Approach,* 3rd ed. St. Louis: C.V. Mosby Co., 1989.

Reiss, B.S., and Evans, M.E. *Pharmacological Aspects of Nursing Care,* 3rd ed. Albany, N.Y.: Delmar Pubs., Inc., 1990.

# SELF-TEST

Test your knowledge and skills at your own pace by answering the multiple-choice questions on pages 209 to 211. Answers appear on page 211.

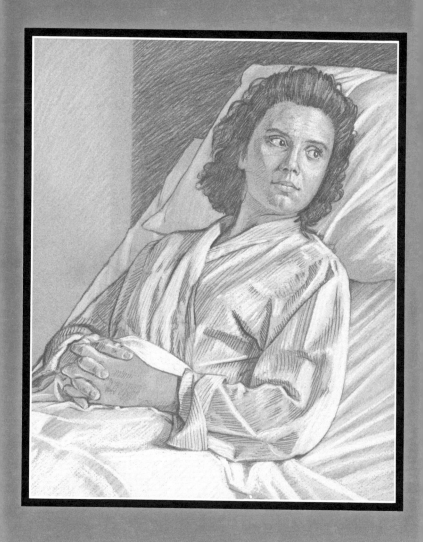

**1.** *Which of the following uses a rating scale to measure the stress caused by significant life events?*
a. Holmes and Rahe's theory
b. the general adaptation syndrome theory
c. the general systems theory
d. Lazarus's theory

**2.** *According to Freud's intrapsychic theory, the id:*
a. tests reality.
b. provides moral judgments.
c. helps solve problems.
d. acts instinctively.

**3.** *When a person has a strong impulse to act in a socially unacceptable manner but substitutes acceptable behavior, he's:*
a. regressing.
b. projecting.
c. dissociating.
d. sublimating.

**4.** *When you enter 54-year-old Mrs. Fenton's room, she greets you like a long-lost friend and tells you how nice you look. She talks constantly while you check her chart, flattering you the whole time. What type of manipulative behavior is she demonstrating?*
a. disparaging maneuvers
b. distracting maneuvers
c. aggressive maneuvers
d. self-destructive maneuvers

**5.** *An aggressive patient tells you he's frustrated because he has to wait for his treatment. You say to him, "Yes, I agree with you; it's uncomfortable to have to wait so long for your treatment." Which "talk down" technique are you using?*
a. dislocation of expectation
b. overdosing
c. de-escalation
d. clarification

**6.** *A patient who deliberately feigns or exaggerates his symptoms for ulterior motives is:*
a. exhibiting obsessive-compulsive behavior.
b. exhibiting aggressive behavior.
c. exhibiting noncompliant behavior.
d. malingering.

**7.** *Which of the following can help in the long-term management of a phobia?*
a. behavioral techniques
b. desensitization
c. social skills training
d. positive reinforcement

**8.** *Cognitive therapy involves:*
a. relaxation.
b. visualization.
c. thought stopping.
d. deep breathing.

**9.** *When you tell Mr. Bergman he'll be moving to a room on the top floor of the hospital, he becomes extremely anxious and asks not to be moved "so high up." You'd suspect that he has:*
a. acrophobia.
b. glossophobia.
c. agoraphobia.
d. claustrophobia.

**10.** *In response to anxiety, the sympathetic nervous system produces cardiovascular effects, including:*
a. fainting.
b. decreased blood pressure.
c. increased heart rate.
d. decreased pulse rate.

**11.** *In response to anxiety, the parasympathetic nervous system produces neuromuscular effects, including:*
a. nausea.
b. loss of appetite.
c. an aversion to food.
d. abdominal discomfort.

**12.** *Confusion that has a rapid onset and results from a reversible physical condition is called:*
a. organic brain syndrome.
b. dementia.
c. delirium.
d. Alzheimer's disease.

**13.** *Dementia can stem from:*
a. oxygen deprivation.
b. an acid-base imbalance.
c. drug intoxication.
d. a central nervous system infection.

**14.** *When talking to a depressed patient, which of the following statements would you use to initiate therapeutic communication?*
a. "You'll feel better soon."
b. "Don't dwell on your problems."
c. "Don't feel like that."
d. "You look upset. Tell me what you're thinking."

**15.** *Therapeutic serum levels for lithium range from:*
a. 0.5 to 1 mEq/liter.
b. 0.8 to 1.2 mEq/liter.
c. 1 to 2 mEq/liter.
d. 2 to 3 mEq/liter.

**16.** *Unresolved grief commonly causes:*
a. violent behavior.
b. mild, chronic depression.
c. an increase in food and alcohol consumption.
d. an increase in physical activities.

**17.** *To help a patient and his family through the grieving process, you should first:*
a. examine your own feelings about death and dying.
b. encourage them to express their fears.
c. encourage them to express their anger.
d. examine their religious background.

**18.** *To help a grieving patient cope, which of the following statements would you use?*
a. "Try to keep busy."
b. "Don't be sad."
c. "You must feel a tremendous loss."
d. "Life will go on."

**19.** *Which of the following is an adaptive reaction to grief?*
a. suppression
b. mourning
c. denial
d. repression

**20.** *In patients with schizophrenia, hallucinations usually occur during the:*
a. active phase.
b. prodromal phase.
c. acute phase.
d. residual phase.

**21.** *Dysfunctional thought form causes:*
a. delusions.
b. loose associations.
c. thought broadcasting.
d. thought insertion.

**22.** *In schizophrenia, which type of hallucination occurs most commonly?*
a. olfactory
b. tactile
c. auditory
d. visual

**23.** *The most common characteristic of schizophrenia is:*
a. a flattened or blunted affect.
b. loose associations.
c. hallucinations.
d. a psychomotor disturbance.

**24.** *Once a patient has been placed in restraints, you should monitor him every:*
a. 5 minutes.
b. 15 minutes.
c. 30 minutes.
d. 60 minutes.

**25.** *Antipsychotic drugs cause:*
a. moderate sedative and anticholinergic effects and a moderate incidence of extrapyramidal symptoms.
b. minimal sedative and anticholinergic effects and a high incidence of extrapyramidal symptoms.
c. strong sedative and anticholinergic effects and a low incidence of extrapyramidal symptoms.
d. strong sedative and weak anticholinergic effects and a high incidence of extrapyramidal symptoms.

**26.** *As you examine a psychotic patient, you note that he keeps repeating the same phrase over and over. This form of altered communication is known as:*
a. echolalia.
b. perseveration.
c. circumstantial speech.
d. tangential speech.

**27.** Medical management of an anorexic patient aims to prevent a decrease in body weight of more than:
a. 5%.
b. 10%.
c. 15%.
d. 20%.

**28.** Which of the following is a significant sign of bulimia?
a. dental caries
b. irregular menses
c. amenorrhea
d. excessive exercise

**29.** Which of the following can decrease urine specific gravity in a bulimic patient?
a. fasting
b. dehydration
c. water loading
d. weight loss

**30.** To measure skinfold thickness in a man, you'd use:
a. his triceps, abdomen, and thigh.
b. his chest, abdomen, and thigh.
c. his chest, suprailium, and thigh.
d. his triceps, suprailium, and thigh.

**31.** What's the approximate age of a bruise that has turned green?
a. 0 to 2 days
b. 2 to 5 days
c. 5 to 7 days
d. 10 to 14 days

**32.** The first thing you should do for a patient who's been abused or neglected is:
a. relieve his stress.
b. provide him with a safe environment.
c. give him emotional support.
d. treat the physical consequences of the abuse or neglect.

**33.** A victim suffering from rape trauma syndrome will most likely seek counseling and support during the:
a. acute phase.
b. denial phase.
c. reorganizational phase.
d. outward adjustment phase.

**34.** Which of the following psychoactive drugs is not addictive?
a. antianxiety agents
b. stimulants
c. hallucinogens
d. central nervous system depressants

**35.** Constricted pupils may result from:
a. opiate withdrawal.
b. hallucinogen use.
c. amphetamine use.
d. hallucinogen withdrawal.

**36.** When assessing an acutely intoxicated patient, you should do all of the following except:
a. approach him in a nonthreatening manner.
b. maintain constant eye contact.
c. keep listening to him despite verbal abuse.
d. ask other staff members for help if the patient becomes aggressive.

**37.** To prevent a reaction during disulfiram therapy, advise your patient to avoid:
a. aspirin.
b. coffee.
c. tea.
d. after-shave lotion.

**38.** Teach a recovering alcoholic to avoid over-the-counter medications that have an alcohol content of more than:
a. 0.5%.
b. 1.5%.
c. 2.8%.
d. 3.8%.

**ANSWERS**

| | | | | | | | |
|---|---|---|---|---|---|---|---|
| **1.** a | **6.** d | **11.** a | **16.** b | **21.** b | **26.** b | **31.** c | **36.** b |
| **2.** d | **7.** b | **12.** c | **17.** a | **22.** c | **27.** c | **32.** d | **37.** d |
| **3.** d | **8.** c | **13.** d | **18.** c | **23.** a | **28.** a | **33.** c | **38.** d |
| **4.** b | **9.** a | **14.** d | **19.** b | **24.** b | **29.** c | **34.** c | |
| **5.** b | **10.** c | **15.** b | **20.** a | **25.** b | **30.** b | **35.** a | |

# INDEX

**213**

# INDEX

**A**

Abuse. *See also* Rape *and*
  Substance abuse.
  of child, 165-171
  of elders, 176-179
  misconceptions about, 164-165
  of spouse, 172-176
  types of, 163-164
Abusive man, characteristics of, 174
Abusive parent, characteristics of, 170
Acute alcohol intoxication
  assessment of, 189-190
  interventions for, 202-203
Acute drug intoxication
  assessment of, 193, 199
  interventions for, 204-205
Adverse drug reactions, recognizing, 28
Aggressive patient, 41-48
  assessment of, 41-44
  causes of behavior in, 43-44
  evaluating effectiveness of interventions
    for, 46, 48
  interventions for, 44-46, 47
Alcohol abuse
  assessment of, 190-193
  characteristics of patients with, 187
  interventions for, 197t, 203-204
  signs of, 197t
Alcohol levels, effect of, on behavior, 191
Alcohol screening test, 192
Alcohol withdrawal, 193
  delirium and, 193
  signs of, 194
Amitriptyline hydrochloride, 104, 152t
Amoxapine, 104, 152t
Amphetamines
  abuse of, 195t
  as treatment for obesity, 159
Anorexia nervosa, 142, 144-149
  assessment of, 144-145, 147
  criteria for diagnosing, 142
  eating patterns in, 144, 145
  evaluating effectiveness of interventions
    for, 148
  hospitalization for, 147
  interventions for, 147-149
Antianxiety agents
  adverse reactions to, 28
  commonly prescribed types of, 74
  as treatment for confusion, 87
Anticipatory grief, 111
Antidepressants
  administration of, 104-105
  adverse reactions to, 28
  as treatment for bulimia, 152, 152t
  types of, 103
Antimanics, adverse reactions to, 28

Antipsychotic drugs, 136-138
  adverse effects of, 28, 137-138
  types of, 137
Anxiety, 61-77
  aggression and, 68
  assessment of, 67-69
  body's response to, 64i
  evaluating patient with, 76
  family relationships and, 68-69
  immediate interventions for, 69-73
  long-term management of, 73-76
  pathologic, 61
  physical disorders associated with, 66
  psychophysiologic effects of, 63, 65
  signs of, 67-68
  theories on, 65-67
  triggers for, 69
  types of, 61-62
Anxiolytics. *See* Antianxiety agents.
Ascendin, 104, 152t
Assessment of psychosocial crises, 11,
  13, 19-31

**B**

Barbiturate abuse, 198t
Battered spouse. *See* Spouse abuse.
Benzocaine, as treatment for obesity, 159
Benzodiazepine abuse, 197t
Bereaved family, coping of, 120
Binge eating, 150
Body types, obesity and, 155, 156i
Borderline personality disorder, psychosis
  and, 128
Bruise, estimating age of, 167t
Bulimia nervosa, 143, 149-153
  assessment of, 150-152
  criteria for diagnosing, 143
  evaluating effectiveness of interventions
    for, 153
  interventions for, 152-153
Bulk fillers, as treatment for obesity, 159
Bupropion, 105

**C**

Cannabinoid abuse, 199t
Chemical use, psychosis and, 129
Child abuse, 165-171
  assessment of, 165-170
  characteristics of parent responsible
    for, 170
  evaluating effectiveness of interventions
    for, 171
  interventions for, 170-171
  risk factors for, in family, 169
  support groups for, 166
  types of, 168
Cocaine abuse, 195t

*i* refers to an illustration; *t* refers to a table

Cognitive theory of stress response, 5
Communication, nurse-patient, 19-22
  barriers to, 20, 22
  nonverbal, 19
  techniques of, 19, 21
Competence
  assessing, 16
  informed consent and, 15
Compulsions, 53. *See also* Obsessive-
    compulsive patient.
Confusion, 79-88
  assessment of, 80-83, 84, 85t
  coping with patient with, 87
  evaluating effectiveness of interventions
    for, 88
  interventions for, 83, 85
Conversion disorder, 51
Coping strategies for stress
  assessment of, 11, 13
  types of, 5, 9, 30

**D**
Delirium. *See also* Confusion.
  assessment of, 82
  causes of, 79
  criteria for diagnosing, 81
  vs. dementia, 82t
Dementia. *See also* Confusion.
  assessment of, 83
  causes of, 79-80
  criteria for diagnosing, 81
  vs. delirium, 82t
  determining severity of, 88
Dependent patient, 56-59
  assessment of, 57
  characteristic behavior of, 56-57
  evaluating effectiveness of interventions
    for, 58-59
  interventions for, 58
Depressant abuse, 197t
Depression, 91-108
  assessment of, 97-100
  behavioral symptoms in, 99
  care plan for patient with, 101-102t
  causes of, 95-97
  criteria for diagnosing, 108
  interventions for, 100-107
  patients at risk for, 93-95
  suicide risk in, 98, 99-100
  types of, 91-93
DES. *See* Diethylstilbestrol.
Desipramine hydrochloride, 104, 152t
Desyrel, 105, 152t
Diagnostic tests, 30-31
Diethylstilbestrol, 183
Documentation of psychosocial crises, 16
Domestic abuse, 163
Doxepin hydrochloride, 104
Drug abuse
  assessment of, 200-202
  characteristics of patient with, 187-188
  interventions for, 205-207

Drug-alcohol interactions, 190t
Dysfunctional thoughts, 126

**EF**
Eating attitudes test, 146
Eating disorders, 141-160. *See also* An-
    orexia nervosa *and* Bulimia nervosa.
  adolescents and, 149
  causes of, 141-143
  incidence of, 141
  patient care challenges in, 143
  prevalence of, 141
  types of, 141
Elavil, 104, 152t
Elder abuse, 176-179
  assessment of, 176-177
  causes of, 176
  evaluating effectiveness of interventions
    for, 179
  interventions for, 178-179
Electroconvulsive therapy, 107
Emotional abuse, 163
Environmental manipulation
  anxiety and, 70-71
  confused patient and, 86
Evaluation of psychosocial crises, 13-14
Fetal alcohol syndrome, 193
Fight-or-flight response, 68
Fluoxetine, 105

**GH**
General adaptation syndrome theory of
    stress response, 3-4, 6-7
Generalized anxiety disorders, 62
Goldfarb's scale for evaluating cognitive
    impairment, 84
Grief, 111-121
  assessment of, 116-118
  evaluating effectiveness of interventions
    for, 121
  interventions for, 118-119, 121
  responses to, 111-115
    adaptive vs. maladaptive, 114-115
  stages of, 113t
  types of, 111
  unresolved, 114-116, 117-118
Hallucinogen abuse, 196t
Holmes and Rahe's theory of stress re-
    sponse, 4
Hyperventilation, treatment of, 71-72

**IJK**
Imipramine hydrochloride, 104i
Informed consent, 14-15
Interpersonal theory of stress response, 5
Intervention for psychosocial crises, 13
Interviewing patient, 22-27, 29-30
Intrapsychic theory of stress response, 5
Isocarboxazid, 105

**L**
Lazarus's theory of stress response, 4

*i* refers to an illustration; *t* refers to a table

Legal issues, psychosocial crisis and, 14-16
Lithium, as treatment for manic-depressive illness, 103, 108
Ludiomil, 105
Lysergic acid diethylamide (LSD) abuse, 196t

M
Major depression, 91-92
    criteria for diagnosing, 92
    psychosis and, 128
Malingering patient, 50-52
    assessment of, 51-52
    evaluating progress of, 52
    interventions for, 52
Malingering vs. psychological disorders, 51
Manic-depressive illness, 92-93
Manic episode
    criteria for diagnosing, 94
    psychosis and, 128
Manipulative patient, 33-38
    assessment of, 34-35
    characteristic behaviors of, 34
    evaluating effectiveness of interventions for, 37-38
    interventions for, 35-37
    maneuvers used by, 34-35
    manipulation cycle and, 36
    setting limits on behavior of, 35-36, 37
Maprotiline hydrochloride, 105
Marijuana abuse, 199t
Marplan, 105
Memory loss, assessment of, 83
Mental illness vs. psychosocial crisis, 4
Mental status examination, 23, 24, 26-27
Monoamine oxidase (MAO) inhibitors, 103, 105
Münchausen syndrome, 51

N
Nardil, 105
Neglect, 163-164
Neuroleptics, 97
Neurologic disorders, psychosis and, 129-130
Noncompliant patient, 38-41
    assessment of, 38-39
    behavioral symptoms of, 38
    collaborating with, 40
    evaluating effectiveness of interventions for, 41
    interventions for, 39-41
Norpramin, 104, 152t
Nortriptyline hydrochloride, 104, 152t
Nurse-patient contract, 40
Nurse-patient manipulation cycle, 36
Nursing diagnoses for psychosocial problems, 12-13
Nursing process, psychosocial crisis and, 11, 13-14

O
Obesity, 153-160
    assessment of, 157
    causes of, 154-155, 157
    classifying, 154
    drug therapy and, 159
    evaluating effectiveness of interventions for, 160
    interventions for, 157-160
    physiologic risks of, 154
    psychological ramifications of, 154
    sleep difficulties and, 154
Obsessions, 52-53. See also Obsessive-compulsive patient.
Obsessive-compulsive disorder, 62
Obsessive-compulsive patient, 52-56
    assessment of, 53, 54
    behavioral symptoms of, 52-53, 54
    evaluating effectiveness of interventions for, 56
    interventions for, 54-56
Opiate abuse, 198t

PQ
Pamelor, 104, 152t
Panic disorders, 62
Parnate, 105
Patient's rights, 15
Phencyclidine abuse, 196t
Phenelzine sulfate, 105
Phenylpropanolamine, as treatment for obesity, 159
Phobias, 62
Physical abuse, 163
Planning for psychosocial crises, 13
Postoperative psychosis, 129
Postpartum depression, 98
Posttraumatic stress disorder, 62
    psychosis and, 128
Protriptyline hydrochloride, 104
Prozac, 105
Psychological disorders vs. malingering, 51
Psychotic disorders, 123-139
    assessment of, 130-134
    behavioral characteristics in, 131-133
    causes of, 128-130
    challenges in caring for patients with, 130
    evaluating effectiveness of interventions for, 138-139
    interventions for, 134, 136-138
    physical disorders that cause signs of, 129
    preventing assault in, 135
    psychotic crisis in, 133
    restraining patient with, 134
    safety concerns in, 133-134
    schizophrenia, as type of, 123-128
    speech dysfunctions in, 132
    symptom triggers in, 131

*i* refers to an illustration; *t* refers to a table

**R**
Rape, 179-184
  assessment of, 179-182
  easing patient distress in, 182
  evaluating effectiveness of interventions
      for, 184
  interventions for, 182-184
  male victims of, 181
Rape-trauma syndrome, 180t
Referential thinking, 126
Relaxation techniques, 71, 72
Restraints
  application of, 45-46
  caring for patient in, 47
  types of, 46
  use of, 16-17
    during psychotic episode, 134

**S**
Schizophrenia, 123-128. *See also* Psy-
      chotic disorders.
  criteria for diagnosing, 124
  incidence of, 123
  phases of, 124-126
  theories on causes of, 126-128
  types of, 124, 125
Seasonal affective disorder, 92
Sexual abuse, 163
Sexually inappropriate behavior, 48-50
  assessment of, 48-49
  dealing with, 50
  evaluating effectiveness of interventions
      for, 50
  forms of, 48
  interventions for, 49-50
  underlying factors in, 48-49
Sinequan, 104
Social readjustment rating scale, 8
Somatization disorder, 51
Spouse abuse, 172-176
  assessment of, 172-173
  characteristics of man responsible for,
      174
  evaluating effectiveness of interventions
      for, 175-176
  interventions for, 173-175
  planning ahead to escape, 175
Stimulant abuse, 195t

Stress
  coping with, 5, 9
  effects of, 2-3
  hospitalized patient and, 3
  theories on response to, 3-7, 9
Substance abuse, 186-207
  assessment of, 189-194, 200-202
  causes of, 188-189
  characteristics of patients with, 186-188
  criteria for diagnosing, 187
  evaluating effectiveness of interventions
      for, 207
  interventions for, 202-207
  patient care challenges in, 188
  support groups for, 206
Suicide
  assessing potential for, 98, 99-100
  preventing, 107
Surmontil, 104

**TU**
Talk-down techniques for aggressive pa-
      tient, 44-45
Therapeutic communication
  anxiety and, 69-70
  confused patient and, 85-86
  depressed patient and, 100, 102-103
  grieving patient and, 118-119
Therapeutic relationship, establishing, 19,
      20
Thought blocking, 126, 132
Thought broadcasting, 126
Thought insertion, 126
Tofranil, 104
Tranylcypromine sulfate, 105
Trazodone hydrochloride, 105, 152t
Trimipramine maleate, 104

**V**
Violence, risk factors for, 43
Violent behavior, stages of, 42
Vivactil, 104

**WXYZ**
Weapon, guidelines for patient with, 45
Weight chart, 148
Wellbutrin, 105